Hoosier Home
Remedies

*Good Health
and
Good Reading
for Della Willman,*

Varo E. Tyler

HOOSIER HOME REMEDIES

Compiled and Considered
by
Varro E. Tyler

Purdue University Press
West Lafayette, Indiana

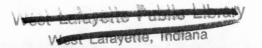

Book and jacket design
by Eileen Butz
Book and jacket photographs
by David Umberger

Published 1985

3/89 gift

Library of Congress Cataloging in Publication Data

Tyler, Varro E.
    Hoosier home remedies.
    Bibliography: p.
    Includes index.
    1. Folk medicine—Indiana—Formulae, receipts, prescrip-
tions.   2. Materia medica, Vegetable—Indiana.   I. Title.
GR110.I6T95 1985   615.8'82771   85-9515
ISBN 0–911198–77–6

Printed in the United States of America

This one's for Jeanne and David

Table of Contents

viii

⟿ Acknowledgments ⟿

More than 175 individuals participated in the preparation of this book. Their contributions were both direct and indirect, that is, through personal or telephone conversations, written correspondence, publications, or participation in such projects as those sponsored by the Indiana University Folklore Archives or in the Indiana Extension Homemakers Association Oral History Project, the records of which were kindly made available to me. I wish to express my sincere thanks to all of these individuals whose names appear in the list of contributors for their assistance in preserving this significant sampling of old Hoosier home remedies for future generations.

In addition, thanks are due to Richard P. Smith of the University News Service, Purdue University, for helping publicize throughout the State of Indiana my desire for information on folk remedies. Also, thanks to James P. Fenn who spent much time searching various archives for me, to Linda Michael and Virginia Tyler who patiently typed and retyped the manuscript, to George R. Spratto who carefully checked the comments on the various remedies for pharmacologic and therapeutic accuracy, to President Steven C. Beering and Provost Felix Haas of Purdue University who graciously allowed me to take a sabbatical leave from my administrative and educational responsibilities in order to write this book, to Prof. Dr. Albrecht Jungk whose invitation to spend six months at the Institut für Agrikulturchemie, Universität Göttingen in Germany gave me time to do so, and, finally, to Adelbert M. Knevel who made it possible by assuming my duties at Purdue during this period.

To all of these and to others who contributed in any way, I express my heartfelt appreciation!

⇒ Contributors ⇐

Ben Alkire
Theodora Andrews
Anonymous
Eleanor Arnold
Marge Aughenbaugh
Mrs. Tom Bailey
Mrs. Woodrow Barker
Mrs. Walter B. Bates
Cledia Bertke
Madge Ellett Bloomfield
Virgie Rowles Bowers
Inez Bowyer
Richard W. Brandon
Eva Brandt
Paul G. Brewster
Margaret Brown
Mary Ann Brown
Evelyn Buchanan
Susan Buriak
Carol Burke
Ruby Stainbrook Butler
Richard Carter
Mrs. Chapel
David Chesak
Ola B. Chillson
Henry Chopson
Claudia Otten Clark
Helen Clawson
Sarah W. Coleman
Jane Cowgill
Martha Crail
George Davidson
N. Davidson
Ruby Dawson
Charles C. Deam
Mildred Dively
Eva K. Doty
Lina Bell Duncan
Blanche Duzan
Sandra Earnest
Ethel Ellett
Madge Ellett
Nelda Ellis
Anna Evans

Judith Fehrmann
Florence Field
Vonda Fiscus
Barbara Fluegeman
Margie M. Fogleman
Mary Fouts
Thelma B. Fox
Chester A. Garner
Hazel Garrett
Margaret Garrison
Pearl Garrison
James Gatska
Sylvia P. Gibbons
Emily Gilotti
Mrs. Charles Glasson
Mary (Molly) Gleason
Marta Goris
Ruth J. Grant
Dee Grose
Beulah Grinstead
Violetta Halpert
Esther M. Halter
Mrs. Dale William Hamilton
Ella Harbaugh
Loretta Hatfield
Grace Hawkins
Josephine Hayes
Florence Henchman
Sue Henderson
Pearl Mutchler Hilard
Dorothy Hoffman
Mrs. Wayne Hollen
Lillian Hoover
John Edward Hopkins
Juanita Hunter
Mrs. Marshall Huntzinger
Clarence G. Hurley
Lucile M. Imes
Mrs. Jackson
Mrs. Fred Jeide
Ethel W. Johnson
Mrs. Hershel Johnson
Charles Jones
Joyce M. Kelley

Carolyn Kellum
Betty Kingston
Edith M. Kistler
Mary Klarke
Edna Mae Klinstiver
Betty Krieg
Carol V. Lamb
Irene Lankford
Julia Koch LaSelle
Edward S. Lauterbach
Dorris B. Layman
Philip R. LeGrand
Helen Lombardo
Shaunn Lybarger
James "Luke" Mann
Karen McCoy
Carmelita McGurk
Mary Elizabeth McKnight
Ruth McNabb
Etta McNeely
Mrs. Walter W. Miskus
Peggy Ann Moore
Mary B. Moorman
Ada Mullis
Maude Nellis
Betty Nelson
Elizabeth Newby
Carol Newman
Mrs. Charles Newman
Jennie Niendorf
Rose Nisenbaum
Edna S. Northerner
Bert Ogborn
William E. Osborne
Doris Parks
Helen Patrick
Marsha A. Patterson
Mrs. Leslie Peters
George Piranian
Edwin D. Posey
Beulah Ramey
Glenn Richardson
Rachel Road

Warren E. Roberts
Oliver W. Robinson
Colista Rogers
John Rogula
Mrs. Lani Rosenberger
Lillian N. Rosner
Dorothy Rowley
Essie Marie Rumble
Sylvia Schwartz
Mary Ann Seils
S. H. Selman
Bernice Shell
Farel Shuger
Harry Shuger
Sylvia Shuger
Jane Slusser
Helen Smalley
Inez Smith
Millie Smith
Ruby Smith
Mary Stevens
Lucille Sturgeon
W. J. Tallant
Bill Thomas
Joseph D. Tilford
Doris Tilghman
Edna Vandenbark
Stella Vanderhoef
Mrs. Verne Vandivier
Arnold Varney
Mrs. Huber Waggaman
Alice M. Wenger
Alice Whiteford
Jim Whiteford
Mrs. Roscoe Whitezel
Opal Whitsett
Mrs. Earl Wiles
Mary Willets
John R. Williams
Thelma Williams
Charles H. Wininger
Clarence B. Wolfe
Ed Workman

❧❧❧ Foreword ❧❧❧

This volume is a labor of love stemming from one of Dr. Tyler's lifelong hobbies. He covers the medical history of the heartland as seen through our folk remedies, discussing subjects ranging from baldness to athlete's foot. The 81 physical conditions that are listed alphabetically called forth the surprising number of nearly 800 home remedies. Dr. Tyler was assisted in his work by some 175 contributors. His commentaries are especially useful, since they are written in nonmedical terms and nicely complement the catalog of cures.

The lore of home remedies is rich in superstition, ritual, and magic. Fortunately, most of these concoctions and ministrations are harmless, many make good common sense, and some are actually scientifically sound. Most treatments are symptomatic rather than specific. Chicken soup is listed as a cure-all. This treatment has certainly stood the test of time. In fact, the venerable Mount Sinai Hospital of New York is now selling canned chicken soup in its gift shop. And when all else fails, you can always "hang your hat on a bedpost and drink whiskey until you see two hats."

Steven C. Beering, MD, FACP
President, Purdue University

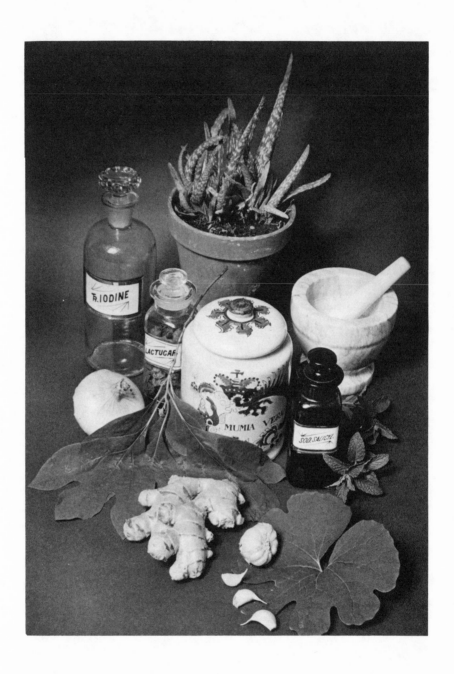

Introduction

No single state is more typical of the entire United States than is Indiana. When movie producers want to designate an All-American hero-type, they wisely select the name Indiana Jones. When sociologists want to study the inhabitants of a typical American town, Muncie, Indiana, becomes the area to undergo scrutiny. From the heavily industrialized northwest "region" to the fertile plains of its central farmland to the rolling, wooded hills of its picturesque southern reaches, Indiana is indeed America in miniature.

What is true of the land is also true of its people. The original Indian mound builders; the later Miami, Delaware, and Shawnee, among others; the French trappers and traders; the early American pioneers and later settlers from the eastern states; the Old World immigrants who either settled there or passed through; all combined to make Indiana the most American of the United States of America.

Many of the inhabitants of the state which came to be known as "the crossroads of the nation" possessed a rich heritage of practical information about the prevention and cure of disease. Passed down to them from all of these forebears, the remedies utilized readily available materials ranging from the abundant wild plants to common household products such as laundry soap and kerosene. Because of the diverse nature of the state and its people, these Hoosier home cures are, in fact, a representative selection of American folk medicine. For this reason, it became important to record the remedies while information concerning their formulation and preparation was still present in the minds of those who originally learned them from their mothers, grandmothers, and great-grandmothers. Home doctoring was, in the past, typically "women's work."

Widespread publicity concerning this project brought literally scores of letters from Hoosiers (mostly female, many of them elderly) listing their favorite remedies. A few originated from individuals in neighboring states, especially Illinois, Kentucky, and Ohio; these, too, were included in the belief that knowledge is not rigidly contained by man-made boundaries. The few previously published articles and books on the subject were scrutinized, as were the appropriate sections of the files of the Folklore Archives of Indiana University. The Indiana Extension Homemakers Association Oral History Project also con-

1

tributed useful information. From all of these individual and collective sources, whose names are acknowledged elsewhere, came the information which makes up this volume.

The remedies are organized according to the disease state or ailment for which they are recommended. Sequence is approximately alphabetical according to the principal ingredients. These appear as headings to the individual remedies in order to facilitate a rapid scanning of, especially, the longer listings. In the case of herbal remedies, the correct botanical name of all except the most common spices and vegetables is given in addition to the common name supplied by the informant. However, to avoid unnecessary complexity of little interest or value to most readers, the author citation is not included as part of the scientific name. The correct name with author citation appears together with appropriate synonyms in the appendix. *Flora of Indiana* by Charles C. Deam, Department of Conservation, Division of Forestry, Indianapolis, 1940, 1,236 pages, was used as the primary botanical authority for both the popular and scientific names of Indiana plants.

Because so many of the remedies were supplied by numerous informants—ten different people described the use of an onion poultice to treat colds and flu—the names of persons are not recorded in connection with specific cures. Occasionally, an interesting or useful comment is noted with the name of the contributor. These appear in italics rather than in quotation marks since, in many cases, I have recorded them in a slightly modified form for the sake of clarity or brevity. In no case has the meaning itself been changed.

More than 750 Hoosier folk medicines are included in this book. The list could have been much longer, but many were purposely excluded. Folk remedies are a curious mixture of sense and nonsense. Although it is often difficult to separate completely the two categories because of the paucity of scientific study devoted to this field, cures obviously dependent upon magic, myth, and superstition were eliminated. Literally dozens of "cures" for warts fall into this class. Perhaps the most frequently reported magical remedy involves carrying a buckeye or horse chestnut in the pocket to prevent and cure rheumatism and arthritis. This is a very widely held belief of ancient European origin.

On the other hand, a very few recipes to alleviate hunger and thirst are included, along with such miscellaneous items as an insect repellant for horses as well as people and a method of rendering fish bait more attractive. Although these do not deal strictly with medical problems, they seemed sufficiently interesting to merit listing.

Nature is said to resist classification, and natural remedies are no exception. I found it particularly difficult to draw arbitrary lines between treatments for colds and flu in comparison to those intended for coughs and croup or for sore throat. Nevertheless, since each of these three categories is a relatively large one comprising 61, 36, and 23 remedies, respectively, it seemed useful to categorize them as precisely as possible instead of grouping them all together. Similar problems were encountered with the categories dealing with burns; cuts, bruises, and abrasions; wounds; and wounds, cuts, burns, sprains, sores, etc. Classification in all cases is strictly according to the statements of the informants.

Some of the information supplied by correspondents and informants was particularly surprising even to the compiler who possesses more than thirty years' experience in dealing with natural-product remedies of all kinds. I was prepared to receive numerous recommendations from Hoosiers for sassafras tea as a "blood thinner" and spring tonic (and I did), but I was completely unprepared to find onions used in every conceivable form, both internally and externally, for practically every condition ranging, alphabetically, from arthritis to wounds. Indeed, based upon the reports I received, onions and, to a lesser extent, their near relative garlic, deserve to be designated as the universal Hoosier remedies.

The frequency with which remedies for particular conditions were submitted gives some idea of the relative significance of those illnesses to people both in the past and in the present. However, just because the number of recipes for treating colds and flu far outnumber those submitted for curing cancer, it does not necessarily follow that the former were more important than the latter. It does indicate that colds and flu were more easily recognized than cancer by laymen and, further, were considered more amenable to home treatment. Also, in considering the number of different cures, it is necessary to keep in mind that some of the more popular ones were submitted by half-a-dozen or more informants, but in the following summary, each different one is counted but once.

Remedies for colds and flu far outnumber all others with 61 different ones recorded; coughs and croup brought 36; stomachache and colic, also 36; various tonics number 32; arthritis and rheumatism cures, 28; burns (including sunburn), 25; wounds, 24; sore throat, 23; diarrhea and dysentery, 22; and poison ivy and poison sumac dermatitis treatments count 21.

Not far behind are remedies for tooth and gum problems—mostly toothache—at 20; boils and carbuncles, and insect bites and sting cures each list 18; sprains and sore muscles, also 18; and headache treatments and kidney problems each number 17.

At the other end of the scale, only a single remedy was provided for gout (there was probably little high living among the Hoosier pioneers), and a single remedy for the tobacco-chewing habit was also submitted, probably because few were interested in breaking the habit. Likewise, perspiration odor, dealt with by one correspondent, was apparently not considered to be much of a problem.

There were several reasons for compiling this list of Hoosier home remedies. They are, of course, of historical interest, and in our present circumstances which rely so heavily on sophisticated medical treatment provided by highly trained physicians, the number of persons who use folk cures, or who even have knowledge of them, is rapidly declining. It was worthwhile to record them, therefore, before all of that knowledge was lost.

But even more important to the author is the belief that among the remedies are at least a few that were used, and that continue to be used, because they were truly effective. Some of the most significant drugs in use today—morphine from the opium poppy, digoxin from the foxglove, ergotamine from the ergot fungus—were discovered as a result of observing the beneficial effects of ancient folk remedies. There is every reason to believe that additional medicines of equal or even greater importance await discovery in other remedies long used but little investigated, at least from the scientific viewpoint.

For this, and for other reasons as well, I have provided brief commentaries on some of the remedies in the various categories. Several of the cures need to be studied more extensively, and this has been noted. Others should not be used as recommended by the informant, not simply because they are without value but because some of them are downright harmful. This, too, has been noted, at least in the more serious cases. As a matter of fact, it is probably imprudent to use any of the remedies listed for the condition indicated, unless one has certain knowledge of its safety and efficacy.

With these brief introductory statements, we can now proceed to the remedies themselves. It is my hope that the lay reader will find them interesting as a study in Hoosier folklore and the scientific reader will find a few of them potentially valuable in providing more effective cures for some of the diseases which have long afflicted human beings.

❧Arthritis and Rheumatism❧

Angleworm Oil

Angleworm oil, prepared by placing the worms in a glass jar in the sun and allowing them to "melt," is applied to rheumatic or arthritic joints. Then cover with red flannel.

Asparagus

Eat large quantities of asparagus and avoid all acidic foods and drinks to obtain great relief from rheumatism in just a few days.

Balsam Cucumber, Witch Hazel, Wintergreen

Grandma's Arthritis Liniment is made as follows:

Balsam cucumbers (balsam pears) (fruit of *Momordica charantia*)	3 or 4
Alcohol	16 ounces
Witch hazel water	4 ounces
Wintergreen oil	2 ounces

Place all the above ingredients in a quart jar, mix, and let steep for a few weeks. Strain off the liquid.

> *Makes a first-class liniment for arthritis in the joints of the hands and wrists.* Ethel W. Johnson

Bee Stings

To cure rheumatism, let several bees sting the affected part. (Note: Caution! This heroic treatment is certainly not recommended, particularly for those persons allergic to insect stings.)

Black Birch

To prepare a salve for treating rheumatism, obtain some sap from the black birch tree (*Betula lenta*).* Mix with a little lard or vaseline. Massage afflicted joints with it, rubbing in as much as possible. Then apply a thin coating. Repeat this treatment every morning and at bedtime.

Celery

Large amounts of celery, boiled in milk or water, will give relief from the discomfort of rheumatism.

Epsom Salts, Baking Soda, Cream of Tartar

Arthritis is relieved with a mixture prepared from 4 table-spoons of epsom salts, 2 of baking soda, and 1 of cream of tartar. Take 1 teaspoonful of the mixture in a cup of warm water every morning before breakfast.

Figs, Raisins, etc.

The figs, raisins, etc., recipe for neuritis in the section Neuritis and Neuralgia is also recommended by a correspondent for arthritis.

Honey, Vinegar

Drink honey and vinegar to cure arthritis.

Honey, Vinegar, Whiskey

Drink honey, vinegar, and whiskey every morning before breakfast to cure arthritis.

---

*Not found in Indiana. Use the yellow birch (*Betula lutea* var. *macrolepis*) instead.

Lemon Juice

Drink quantities of lemon juice to relieve the pain of arthritis.

Neat's Foot Oil, Kerosene

Rheumatism can be cured by rubbing the affected part with a mixture of half neat's foot oil and half kerosene.

Onions, Molasses

An effective cure for rheumatism is made by steeping 6 large onions in a pint of molasses until a thick syrup is formed. Take every 2 or 3 hours.

and Burdock

A tea of burdock roots or leaves (*Arctium minus*) taken simultaneously with the above remedy will improve the effect of the onion syrup.

Pokeberries

Eat fresh or dried pokeberries (*Phytolacca americana*) to treat arthritis. Start with just a few daily and gradually increase the dose.

Pokeberries

Eat pokeberries (*Phytolacca americana*) for rheumatism.

> *My father was helped by eating the berries.*
> Irene Lankford

Pokeberries, Brandy or Wine

Soak ripe pokeberries (*Phytolacca americana*) in brandy or wine to make a tincture that is a great remedy for all kinds of rheumatism. It should be used freely in such cases.

Pokeberries, Whiskey

Soak pokeberries in whiskey and drink the liquid to cure rheumatism.

Pokeberry Juice

Take one quart of mashed, fresh or fresh frozen, ripe pokeberries (*Phytolacca americana*), add 3 quarts of water, and boil 4 to 6 minutes (depending on strength desired). Strain through a fine sieve or cheesecloth. Add 1 pint of dark Karo syrup to the juice and bring to a boil again. Seal in pint or quart fruit jars as you would canned fruit. Take 1 tablespoonful morning and evening in a little water or milk. Refrigerate juice after opening as it spoils easily.

> *I was practically a cripple when it was recommended to me. I took it reluctantly, but after a few weeks, I was able to climb again. That has been four years, and now I am able to work and run like a youngster.* Arnold Varney

Potash, Camphor

To treat rheumatism, add 1 teaspoonful of pulverized potash (potassium carbonate) and a lump of gum camphor the size of a walnut to a pint of alcohol. Use as a liniment.

Rattlesnake, Whiskey

To cure rheumatism, kill a rattlesnake before it has had a chance to strike. Skin it and dry the remains. When dry, put them in a jug of corn whiskey. Drink the whiskey.

Red Beets

Apply a poultice of grated red beets for inflammatory rheumatism.

> *It worked on my husband.* Mrs. Tom Bailey

Saltpeter, Sulfur, Whiskey

Add saltpeter and sulfur to a bottle of whiskey. Take 2 table-spoonfuls every 4 hours for arthritis.

Snake Oil

For rheumatism, cook a snake and collect the resulting oil. Rub on the affected area.

Solomon's Seal

Solomon's seal root (*Polygonatum* spp.) is used to prepare a tea which is effective against rheumatism and arthritis.

Soya Flour

Substitute soya flour for wheat flour in cooking to help arthritis pain.

Starweed

The leaves of starweed (*Stellaria media*) are soaked in water and applied to the affected area to cure rheumatism.

Willow Bark

Willow bark tea (*Salix* spp.) is drunk to cure rheumatism.

Yarrow

For rheumatism, drink yarrow (*Achillea millefolium*) tea.

Comments

Certainly the most interesting and also the most frequently submitted Hoosier remedy for arthritis and rheumatism is pokeberries. These showy, dark purple berries are recommended in the form of fresh or dried fruits, juice, or as an alcoholic extract, and the comments of numerous correspondents testify to their effectiveness.

Normally, all parts of the mature poke plant are considered toxic. People commonly eat the very young shoots as potherbs, but the wisdom of even this practice may be challenged. Workers throughout a large building where quantities of the root were being milled became ill, and a woman who drank one cup of tea made from the root required hospitalization. The berries are much less poisonous than the root, and some authorities claim they are quite safe to eat.

Scientific studies carried out in Europe seem to indicate that pokeberries may induce a kind of nonspecific stimulation of the human immune system. Much more work needs to be done before this can be verified with certainty or before its relation to relief from the pains of arthritis and rheumatism can be definitely established. However, at present, it appears that there may be some basis in fact for the beneficial effects reported from consuming pokeberries. These presumed benefits must nevertheless be considered carefully in view of the known toxic nature of the plant and, possibly, even its fruit.

The external and internal use of salicylates and analgesic and anti-inflammatory agents in the treatment of arthritic conditions is well-known. This explains the effectiveness of the black birch salve which would contain some methyl salicylate and willow bark tea with its content of salicin (salicyl alcohol glucoside). The wintergreen oil (methyl salicylate) added to the balsam cucumber liniment would serve the same purpose when used externally.

The honey and vinegar treatment for arthritis enjoyed a considerable popularity some years ago when it was recommended by a physician in Vermont in a best-selling book. The burdock tea that is recommended here in conjunction with the onion syrup is an old European favorite for the treatment of rheumatism. There is no evidence supporting the effectiveness of either the honey and vinegar or the burdock tea remedies.

Although not listed for reasons explained in the introduction, the practice of carrying a buckeye or horse chestnut in the pocket to prevent or cure rheumatism or arthritis was probably mentioned as frequently by correspondents as any Hoosier remedy for any condition. This custom is extremely widespread, in spite of the fact that there is nothing to indicate it has any real value.

❧Asthma❧

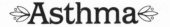

Alfalfa

Alfalfa tea (*Medicago sativa*) will relieve the difficult breathing of a person suffering from asthma.

Honeycomb

Chew a piece of honeycomb to relieve the stuffy feeling of allergy and to help breathing.

> *It gives almost instant relief.* N. Davidson

Hops

Lying on a small pillow filled with hops (*Humulus* spp.) will help one breathe more easily.

Hornet Nest

Drink tea made from a hornet nest to help asthma.

Jack-in-the-Pulpit

Jack-in-the-pulpit root (*Arisaema triphyllum*) will relieve the symptoms of asthma.

Jimson Weed

Smoke the leaves of jimson weed or stramonium (*Datura stramonium*) to relieve asthma.

Jimson Weed, Smooth Sumac

The symptoms of asthma are relieved by smoking a mixture of the leaves of jimson weed (*Datura stramonium*) and of smooth sumac (*Rhus glabra*). The leaves are collected, dried, crumbled, mixed, and smoked in a pipe several times a day and just before retiring.

Mullein

Smoke dried mullein leaves (*Verbascum thapsus*) to relieve the symptoms of asthma.

Mullein

Mullein leaves (*Verbascum thapsus*) are made into a tea which is drunk for asthma and into a poultice which is applied to the chest for breathing problems.

Muskrat Skin

Sufferers from asthma should wear a muskrat skin, fur side down, next to the body over the lungs.

Old-Field Balsam

Dry and smoke old-field balsam (*Gnaphalium obtusifolium*). It loosens up phlegm and is good for asthma attacks because one can cough more easily and get relief.

My sister used this with good results. Josephine Hayes

Saltpeter

To relieve the symptoms of asthma, soak blotting paper in a solution containing about 20% of saltpeter (potassium nitrate) and allow to dry. Burn it at night in the patient's bedroom.

Comments

Jimson weed or stramonium contains several solanaceous alkaloids, principally hyoscyamine and scopolamine, which not only relieve the spasms of the trachea that make breathing difficult during asthma attacks but also reduce the associated respiratory and nasal secretions. The plant is therefore often incorporated in mixtures intended to be burned and the smoke inhaled to relieve such allergic symptoms. The jimson weed and the jimson weed-smooth sumac remedies fall into this category.

Incidentally, commercial products of this type were formerly available for over-the-counter sale in pharmacies. When drug abusers began to employ these products in large quantities to produce a kind of intoxication, the Food and Drug Administration changed the products' status, in 1968, to the prescription drug category. This emphasizes the potential danger associated with the improper use of such powerful remedies.

There is no scientific evidence to support the claims of effectiveness of the other remedies reported in this section. Mullein tea might prove soothing because of its mucilage content as would old-field balsam due to its aromatic properties. The chewing of honeycomb (honey and beeswax) and the drinking of hornet nest tea are particularly interesting—if unproven—recommendations.

❧Athlete's Foot❧

Dog Saliva

To cure athlete's foot, let a dog lick your feet.

Comments

Animal saliva certainly possesses some antiseptic properties as witnessed by the fact that many creatures do lick their wounds to clean them and, apparently, to facilitate healing. Whether dog's saliva possesses sufficient antifungal activity to be effective in the treatment of athlete's foot is, however, open to question.

❧Birth Control❧

Mayapple

Drink tea made from mayapple roots (*Podophyllum peltatum*) to induce abortion.

Pennyroyal

Pennyroyal tea (*Hedeoma pulegioides*) will cause a woman who is in the family way to "come around."

Pennyroyal

Pennyroyal tea (*Hedeoma pulegioides*) was used as a birth-control agent by some Indian tribes.

Sugar, Turpentine

Administer a teaspoonful of sugar saturated with turpentine oil to bring about abortion.

Wild Celeryseed

Wild celeryseed tea (*Apium graveolens*) was also used for birth-control purposes by the Indians.

Comments

Pennyroyal has long had a reputation as an emmenagogue or promoter of the menstrual discharge, but in the popular literature, this term is often used as a euphemism for abortifacient, that is, an agent which produces abortion. While the volatile oil of the plant may indeed cause abortion, it does so only in doses large enough to be fatal or nearly fatal to the consumer. Its use is certainly not recommended.

The root of the mayapple is an extremely potent purgative. Its effect is not restricted to the smooth muscles of the intestinal tract but is also observed on the uterus. For this reason, it may cause abortion, especially if consumed in large amounts.

Turpentine oil and sugar have long had the reputation of being able to induce abortion. The oil does act as an irritant, but it was formerly used internally, in small doses (0.3 milliliter) for various conditions. In large doses, it is quite toxic, causing vomiting, convulsions, shock, etc. The use of it, or of any of the products in this section, for the purpose indicated is not recommended.

⇢Bleeding⇠

Cobweb

Apply cobwebs to stop the flow of blood from injuries or cuts.

Dusty Cobweb

A dusty cobweb is especially good to stop cuts from bleeding.

Flour, Vinegar

Put flour and vinegar paste on a cut to stop the bleeding.

Leather

The scrapings of sole leather applied to a cut will stop bleeding.

Milkweed, Cobweb

Cut the stalk of milkweed (*Asclepias syriaca*) and allow the juice or milk to drip into the cut or wound. Continue to add juice until the bleeding stops. This will work better if applied together with cobwebs.

Puffball

Put the dust (spores) from a puffball (family Lycoperdaceae) on a wound to stop the bleeding.

Puffball, Wild Cherry Gum

For bleeding, put a dried puffball (family Lycoperdaceae) on the wound and seal with gum from a wild cherry tree (*Prunus serotina*).

Sassafras Leaves

An excellent styptic is made by chewing up sassafras leaves (*Sassafras albidum*) until they are very fine and then applying the mass to the wound or cut.

Soot

Pack chimney soot in a cut to stop the bleeding.

Sugar; Salt

Put a little sugar or salt on a cut to stop it from bleeding.

Tea Leaves

Apply wet tea leaves to a cut to stop its bleeding.

Tobacco

A big chew of tobacco applied to a wound will stop it from bleeding.

Yarrow Leaves

Use yarrow leaves (*Achillea millefolium*) to stanch the flow of blood from a cut.

Comments

Methods of stopping bleeding or hemorrhage fall into two basic categories: (1) those which mechanically hinder the flow of blood thereby allowing the body's normal clotting mechanism to function more effectively, and (2) those which act as astringents or styptics and reduce the blood flow by constricting or blocking the severed blood vessels, thus allowing a clot to form. Some treatments combine both functions.

The application of cobwebs (plain or dusty), sugar or salt, soot, and puffball spores, for example, obviously are primarily mechanical treatments. Tea leaves and sole leather scrapings contain astringent tannins and function primarily as styptics. Flour and vinegar paste depends upon the mechanical or physical properties of the flour and the astringency of the vinegar. The combination of cobwebs and milkweed juice (latex) functions in a similar fashion.

⇒Blisters ⇐

Carrots, Plantain, Lard

A good salve for blisters is prepared by scraping or shredding 2 carrots and stirring in 2 tablespoonfuls of lard together with 2 plantain leaves (*Plantago* spp.). When the carrots are well-done, strain, cook, and apply.

Oak Bark

A good remedy for blisters is prepared by boiling oak bark (*Quercus* spp.) in a small amount of water until a strong broth results. Apply locally to blisters.

Comments

Blisters are treated in a fashion similar to burns; indeed, many burns do form blisters, although rubbing or abrasion of the skin is also a frequent cause. The carrot-plantain salve forms a protective fatty-mucilaginous layer on the affected area. Tannin present in the oak-bark broth will precipitate the surface proteins of the blister, forming a coating over it.

⋙Blood Thinners, Purifiers, and Tonics⋘

Burdock Roots

Drink tea made from burdock roots (*Arctium minus*) to thin the blood. A cup is best taken in conjunction with sulfur (1 teaspoonful) and dark molasses (1 teaspoonful).

Catnip, Violets, Rose Hips

Take a fistful of fresh chopped catnip (*Nepeta cataria*), ½ tea-cup of violet flowers (*Viola* spp.) without stems, and ½ eggshell of crushed rose fruits (*Rosa* spp.). Simmer in a quart of water for ½ hour and strain through cloth. Drink cold on hot days and hot on cold days. Add a little sugar if desired. It acts to purify the blood, promotes regularity, soothes nerves, and prevents colds.

The residue may be used as a poultice: hot for headaches, cold for minor burns.

Chamomile

Chamomile tea (*Anthemis nobilis*) is an effective tonic.

Cream of Tartar, Sulfur

A mixture of cream of tartar and sulfur will thin the blood.

Dandelion, Garlic

A healthful spring dish is dandelion greens (*Taraxacum officinale*), either cooked or raw, to which has been added a bit of chopped dandelion root and a clove of garlic.

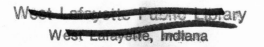

Dandelion, Sarsaparilla

Drink tea made by pouring hot water over equal parts of the dried, pulverized roots of dandelion (*Taraxacum officinale*) and sarsaparilla (*Smilax* spp.). Let stand overnight and use several times the next day. Continue for one month as a helpful tonic for the blood.

Dogwood Bark

The bark of the dogwood tree (*Cornus florida*) is boiled in water to make a bitter tonic.

Garlic

In the spring, eat raw garlic as a tonic.

> *My brother and I both despised it. To this day, I won't even use garlic in cooking.* Pearl Garrison

Gentian

Both the overground plant and the root of gentian (*Gentiana quinquefolia*) are made into a tea that is highly valued as a bitter tonic.

Greens (Mixed)

Mixed greens are eaten as a healthful spring tonic. These consist of young dandelion leaves (*Taraxacum officinale*) cooked with narrow dock (*Rumex crispus*), lamb's quarters (*Chenopodium album*), and wild mustard (*Brassica kaber*). The greens are seasoned with meat fryings and salted to taste.

Herbal Mixture

Collect elecampane root (*Inula helenium*), yellow root (*Hydrastis canadensis*), ginseng (*Panax quinquefolius*), wild cherry bark (*Prunus serotina*), slippery elm bark (*Ulmus fulva*), Solomon's seal (*Polygonatum* spp.), and lobelia (*Lobelia inflata*). After cleaning thoroughly, put them to soak in a quart of brandy until it becomes sufficiently impregnated with the various flavors. Take 1 teaspoonful every day.

> *My grandfather was a temperate man but he*
> *prepared this every spring and took it. He lived*
> *to be past eighty-six.* Eva K. Doty

Honey, Vinegar

Drink 2 teaspoonfuls of honey and 2 of cider vinegar in a glass of water once or twice a day to keep the body functioning smoothly and to prevent almost any illness.

Huckleberries

Make and drink tea from fresh or dried huckleberries (*Gaylussacia baccata*) for an excellent blood purifier and tonic.

Ironwood

Tea made from the wood and/or bark of the ironwood or hop-hornbeam (*Ostrya virginiana*) is drunk as a tonic.

Lavender

The fragrance of lavender flowers (*Lavandula angustifolia*) is inhaled or a tea made from them is drunk to "clear the mind and comfort the spirits."

Poke Shoots

Young poke shoots (*Phytolacca americana*) are cooked and eaten as a spring tonic. The pot liquor in which the greens are cooked is also drunk for the same purpose.

Red Clover

An excellent drink for the blood is strong tea made from the dried blossoms of red clover (*Trifolium pratense*). Use frequently for all blood diseases.

Rock Candy, Cinnamon, Whiskey

Put 1 pound of rock candy and a handful of cinnamon bark into a gallon of good whiskey. Drink as necessary.

> *George Dawson's Receipt for Good Health, September 7, 1873.*

Sassafras

Sassafras root or root-bark tea (*Sassafras albidum*) thins the blood and acts as a tonic.

> *It was good and free.* Ruby Dawson

Sassafras, Honey

Add a teaspoonful of honey to each cup of sassafras tea (*Sassafras albidum*). Drink 1 cup a day in the spring.

Sassafras, Maple Sap

Sassafras root bark (*Sassafras albidum*) in conjunction with heated sugar maple sap (*Acer saccharum*) that has not been cooked down for syrup makes an excellent hot tea for use as a spring tonic. The combination produces an unusual steel-blue colored drink. This was undoubtedly noticed by the very early settlers and led to the use of the inside scrapings of maple bark in making indigo dye.

> *We have used this drink many times to rid ourselves of the late winter blahs.* Barbara Fluegeman

Sassafras

Drink one glass only of sassafras tea (*Sassafras albidum*) as a tonic.

> *Very little is good; too much is bad.* Margie M. Fogleman

Sassafras

Boil sassafras (*Sassafras albidum*) roots or root bark in water to make a beverage which is drunk in the early spring to thin the blood.

Sheep Sorrel

The leaves of sheep sorrel (*Rumex acetosella*) are eaten to produce a feeling of well-being.

Spicewood

Drink tea made from the twigs and leaves of spicewood or spicebush (*Benzoin aestivale*) as a tonic and blood thinner.

Sulfur, Molasses

Take a mixture of sulfur and sorghum molasses to purify the blood in the spring. Repeat several times during the month of March.

Tulip Tree

Tea made from the root bark of the tulip tree (*Liriodendron tulipifera*) is a great tonic. The powdered root bark itself may be taken in small doses once or twice daily. It "operates mildly on the bowels."

> *Used in all weak and debilitated cases of the system.* S. H. Selman

Violet Leaves

Drink violet leaf tea (*Viola* spp.) as a tonic and to "thin the blood" in the spring.

Wild Cherry, Slippery Elm, Whiskey

Wild cherry bark (*Prunus serotina*) and slippery elm bark (*Ulmus fulva*) soaked in whiskey make a good spring tonic.

Wild Strawberry Leaves

The leaves of the wild strawberry (*Fragaria virginiana*), made into a tea, are a useful spring tonic and "blood thinner."

Yellow Dock

Yellow dock tea (*Rumex crispus*) will thin the blood.

Yellow Root

Yellow root tea (*Hydrastis canadensis*) is an effective spring tonic.

Comments

More than twenty different informants recommended the tonic properties of sassafras root (or root bark) tea or a beverage (technically a decoction) made by boiling these plant parts in water. Most mentioned its supposed utility as a "blood thinner" and advised that it be taken in the early spring to modify the blood which had "thickened" during the course of the winter and, in this way, improve the health of the consumer. Only one correspondent expressed caution with respect to the amount to be drunk.

As far as is now known, sassafras has no therapeutically useful properties of any sort. It does not "thin the blood" which likewise does not "thicken" during the winter. Without question, people began to consume it, and many continue to do so, because of its pleasant taste. The practice is nevertheless a hazardous one and cannot be recommended. Sassafras root bark contains a volatile oil which consists of about 80% safrole. Safrole, in turn, has been demonstrated to cause cancer when fed to rats and mice. For this reason, the federal Food and Drug Administration has forbidden the sale of sassafras oil or safrole as flavors or food additives. Root beer, of which sassafras oil was once a main flavoring agent, has not been the same since.

Unfortunately, a great deal of sassafras root bark continues to be collected, sold, made into tea, and drunk. The degree of potential harm of this latter practice is very difficult to determine. It probably presents the same degree of hazard to one's health as cigaret smoking. However, sassafras is supposedly used as a tonic to benefit, not to hurt, the consumer's health. Because it does not do this and because it has no real medicinal value, its use cannot be recommended in spite of its endorsement by many as Indiana's most popular spring tonic.

Some of the other products recommended as tonics are also of interest. Eating fresh greens in the spring no doubt provides certain vitamins, especially A, B_2, C, E, and K, which might have been in short supply during the winter, especially in the age preceding the ubiquitous vitamin pill.

The bitter herbs such as dogwood bark, gentian, and yellow root contained in some recipes have the reputation of stimulating the flow of gastric juices and thereby improving both the appetite and the digestion. They are, therefore, best taken immediately prior to eating.

Chamomile tea is known to possess both antispasmodic and anti-inflammatory properties, thus making it a useful treatment for "what ails you." Likewise, the combination of honey and cider vinegar, thanks to the widely circulated endorsement of a physician in Vermont, is thought to be good for "anything and everything."

Garlic, particularly when eaten raw in quantity, apparently has a beneficial effect on atherosclerosis and high blood pressure and also provides relief from various stomach and intestinal ailments. Unfortunately, consumption of a large clove or so of raw garlic daily is apt to decrease markedly the number of intimate acquaintances of the consumer.

Various tonics prepared by soaking herbs or spices in brandy or whiskey probably rely more upon the temporary stimulating effect and feeling of well-being created by the alcohol than on the medicinal properties of the additives. A vast proprietary-medicine industry was built upon this principle in the latter years of the nineteenth century and continued, in lesser degree, until comparatively modern times.

Sulfur is basically a laxative. It is taken in combination with molasses simply to make it more palatable.

⟪Boils and Carbuncles⟫

Bread, Milk

Treat boils with a poultice of bread and milk, covered with cloth overnight.

Burdock

Apply a poultice made from crushed burdock leaves (*Arctium minus*) to draw out the poison from boils and carbuncles.

Calamus

To treat a carbuncle, boil calamus roots (*Acorus calamus*) until mushy soft, drain, and mash to consistency of mashed potatoes. Spread on a bandage and bind, while still warm, over the carbuncle as a poultice. (Original recipe from Mrs. Peach Sterrett.)

> *My father did this before I retired one night, and the next morning all the corruption went sloughing off. In no time it was well.* Edna S. Northerner

Cornmeal

To cure boils, eat 3 teaspoonfuls of dry cornmeal each morning on arising for 3 days. Do not eat or drink anything prior to the cornmeal. Skip 3 days and repeat, then skip 3 more days and repeat again for a total of 9 teaspoonfuls.

> *By the time I had finished eating the 9 spoon-fuls, the boils had actually dried up. I have never had a boil since.* Henry Chopson

Cornmeal

A cornmeal poultice will cure boils.

Crabgrass

Boils are effectively treated with a crabgrass poultice. This is prepared by cutting up a large handful of crabgrass (*Digitaria sanguinalis*) and moistening in hot water until wilted. Drain, place in a porcelain bowl, add 1 tablespoonful of bacon drippings and ½ cup of salt. Mix well. Place on a clean white cotton cloth and fold in. Place on the boil and leave in place for several hours.

Farina

A boil may be cured by covering it with hot farina.

Fat Meat

A fat meat or salted fat meat poultice will draw the corruption right out of a boil.

Fig

A fig is split open and applied as a poultice to a boil.

Flaxseed

Apply a flaxseed meal poultice to cure boils. It is most effective when hot.

Mud Dauber (Wasp) Nest

Treat boils with a poultice made from a mud dauber nest.

Nutmeg

Eat nutmeg to cure boils.

Onion

To cure a boil, apply the juice from the green stem of an onion.

Onion

Cover the boil with a thick slice of onion and wrap with a cloth to keep the air out and the moisture in.

Peach Tree Leaves

For boils, take peach tree leaves (*Prunus persica*), boil them in water and thicken the resulting liquid with bran. While still warm, pour on a clean thick cloth and hold on the boil.

> *It didn't work very well, We found Unguentine to be of more use in healing boils.* Judith Fehrmann

Potato

To cure a boil, cover with a thick slice of potato and wrap with a cloth to keep the air out and retain moisture.

Suction

Bring a boil to a head by applying suction. A small glass cup is heated with a candle and applied to the skin around the boil. As it cools the matter will be drawn from the boil. Alternatively, drop a strip of lighted paper into a small milk bottle and put the bottle over the boil. This, too, will draw matter out.

Sulfur, Molasses

Take a mixture of sulfur and molasses to prevent boils.

Comments

Boils are basically infections of skin glands by pus-producing organisms. Carbuncles are similar infections of the skin or deeper tissues with multiple openings for the discharge of pus, accompanied by sloughing of dead tissue. Both are commonly treated by the application of materials that are warm, moist, and sometimes fatty to facilitate draining of the pus ("bring to a head") and, ideally, with an accompanying antiseptic action to control the infection.

The poultices or local applications of bread and milk, burdock leaves, calamus, cornmeal, crabgrass, farina, fat meat, figs, flaxseed, mud dauber nest, onions, peach tree leaves, and potatoes, all are treatments of this basic type. They do, no doubt, afford some relief from the accompanying pain of the infection produced by the pressure-causing pus, as does the application of suction which also facilitates drainage. None appears to provide much antiseptic effect.

Eating cornmeal, nutmeg, or the laxative mixture of sulfur and molasses would, as far as we can now say, have little effect on the prevention or treatment of boils. These remedies are, nonetheless, interesting.

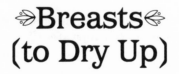

⇢Breasts⇠ (to Dry Up)

Camphor; Turpentine

To dry up the mother's milk after weaning, apply camphor spirits or turpentine oil several times a day to the breasts.

Comments

There is no evidence for the efficacy of either of these products following local application.

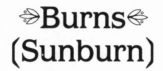

Burns (Sunburn)

Aloe

The fresh juice from an aloe vera plant (*Aloe barbadensis*) will help a burn to heal.

Axle Grease

Apply axle grease to cure a burn.

Baking Soda

Apply baking soda to help heal a burn.

Balm of Gilead Buds

A useful salve for burns is made by boiling balm of gilead buds (*Populus candicans*) in a little water for an hour. Remove the buds and add ½ pound of mutton tallow and ¼ pound of lard to the liquid. Boil until thick.

Blueing

Apply ordinary laundry blueing to heal a burn.

Bread, Milk

Apply a bread and milk poultice to heal a burn.

Butter

To cause a burn to heal quickly, cover it with butter.

Chewing Tobacco

Put a wad of chewing tobacco on a burn to heal it.

Cream

Put pure cream on sunburn to keep it from blistering.

Egg, Flour

Put a mixture of egg and flour on a burn to heal it.

Houseleek

Apply the fresh juice from houseleek or hen and chickens (*Sempervivum tectorum*) to burns. Alternatively, a useful green salve for burns or insect stings can be made by rendering the leaves in lard or a similar fat.

Ice Water

Ice water applied to a burn will relieve the pain quickly.

Kerosene

Dip cotton in kerosene and swab on a burn. It will never blister.

Lard; Fat Meat; Shortening

Put lard, fat meat, or shortening on a burn.

Milkweed

Sunburn is effectively treated with the milk (latex) from milk-weed (*Asclepias syriaca*) diluted half and half with water.

Nightshade

Sunburn is treated by crushing a handful of nightshade leaves (*Solanum nigrum*) and stirring them for a while in a cup of heavy sweet cream. When the cream begins to take on a faint green color from the leaf juices, pat the cream gently on the sunburned area.

Onion Peelings

Bind on onion peelings to help burns heal.

Potato

Put on a slice of raw potato to heal a burn.

Potato

To treat burns, scrape a potato and bind the fine scrapings on the burn with a white cotton cloth.

Potato, Olive Oil, Turpentine

Treat burns or scalds by applying a poultice made from scraped raw potato mixed with sweet oil (olive oil) and a few drops of turpentine spirits. Then cover with honey.

Sedum

The fresh juice from sedum or stonecrop plants (*Sedum* spp.) is a useful treatment for burns and cuts.

Suet

Tie a piece of plain, unrendered suet over a burn, even a severe one, and it will quickly heal.

Tar

For burns, bind on strips of cloth dipped in clean tar.

Tea Leaves

Apply a poultice of tea leaves to stop the pain and help heal burns.

Yellow Prepared Mustard

Yellow prepared mustard is applied directly to a burn to ease the pain and prevent blistering.

Comments

The household treatment of minor burns, scalds, and sunburn depends basically on protecting the exposed tissues with some kind of coating so that the regeneration of new tissues may occur rapidly and without bacterial infection. This is ordinarily done by applying some sort of fatty or mucilaginous coating directly to the affected area. Alternatively, a tannin-containing drug or its equivalent may be applied to precipitate the surface proteins of the exposed area and thus form a mildly antiseptic coating over them.

Fatty materials recommended by informants range from axle grease, to lard or shortening, to cream. They also include various fatty-based ointments containing herbs of a potentially antiseptic nature. Baking soda, eggs and flour, and potato (with its high starch content) tend to form protective layers of a crusty or mucilaginous nature. Tea leaves, rich in tannin, act in the way described above. Ice water not only relieves the pain of minor burns quickly as noted by the informant, it also tends to prevent the formation of blisters.

All of these agents may impede, rather than facilitate, the healing of really serious burns. Such always require professional medical attention.

⇒Cancer⇐

Red Beets

Mash raw red beets to a pulp and apply locally to the external cancer.

Buckeyes

To treat cancer, mash fruits of the buckeye (*Aesculus glabra*), boil until tender, drain, mix with lard, boil again, and allow to cool. Apply the salve locally.

Ear Wax

Apply ear wax locally to cure a cancer.

Garlic, Raisins, Whiskey

To remove a cancerous lump from a woman's breast, add raisins to a pint of whiskey. Then mash up thoroughly 1 handful of garlic and add it to the whiskey, mixing well. Apply this as a plaster to the breast, morning and evening, until the cancer is gone.

Goldenseal

Powdered goldenseal root (*Hydrastis canadensis*) was used by the Indians against all sorts of skin conditions, including, it is said, with great success against cancer.

Pokeweed

Cure a cancer by repeated applications of plasters made from evaporated pokeweed juice (*Phytolacca americana*). After the cancer has been eradicated, heal the remaining ulcer by application of a salve made from equal parts of beeswax, mutton suet, and turpentine spirits melted together.

Red Clover, Narrow Dock

A useful cancer plaster is made by adding 4 handfuls of red clover blossoms (*Trifolium pratense*) to 1 of the roots, or roots and tops, of narrow dock (*Rumex crispus*). Boil in water for some time, strain out the plant parts, and continue careful heating (being very careful not to burn the residue) until it is reduced to the consistency of a salve. Apply as needed.

Red Clover

A product similar to the red clover blossom-narrow dock plaster just described is made with red clover blossoms only (*Trifolium pratense*). Boil several batches in the same water, remove the flowers, and carefully reduce to the consistency of a plaster. Apply by first spreading on a cloth or piece of paper.

Sheep Sorrel (Yellow Wood Sorrel)

Mrs. Brown's Cancer Salve is made as follows:

Collect the largest available stalks of sheep sorrel (*Oxalis stricta*) in August when it produces yellow flowers. Cut off and discard the roots, then pound the blossoms, leaves, and stalks as fine as possible. Put these in a stone crock. If there is not enough juice to keep the plant material moist, add a little water until it can be seen. Let stand 24 hours, then press out all the juice and strain through a clean cloth. Put the juice in a shallow dish or basin and place it in the sun until it thickens into a salve. Keep the salve in a tightly closed tin box or jar so that it will not dry up. For a dry cancer, apply as a plaster 5 or 6 times in 9 days. On the ninth day, the last plaster is removed and the roots of the cancer can be taken out.

I do certify that the above is a receipt in full for the cancer salve, herewith my mark, X, Margaret Brown.

Toad in Butter

To make a salve for cancer, place a toad in a quart of unsalted butter in a sealed can. Set it out in the sun. In a few days, the contents will form an oil which is applied to the cancer.

Pennyroyal, Chamomile, Mullein

For cancer, prepare a salve by boiling pennyroyal (*Hedeoma pulegioides*), chamomile flowers (*Anthemis nobilis*), and mullein (*Verbascum thapsus*) in ½ gallon of apple vinegar for 24 hours. Add salt and 4 ounces of honey; then simmer the mixture down to a salve and apply to the cancer with a feather.

Comments

As far as is now known, none of these recipes has any effectiveness whatever in the treatment of cancer. It would be the height of folly to use any of them and thereby delay seeking competent medical advice for such a condition.

☙Cardiovascular Problems❧

Digitalis

For a weak heart, wash the leaves of the foxglove plant (*Digitalis purpurea*), cut into small pieces, and boil in a small amount of water. Drain and discard the leaves. Add ½ cup of sugar or honey to the juice. Cool and store in a bottle. (Make fresh every 3 days.) Take a teaspoonful every morning.

Garlic, Onions

For high blood pressure, eat garlic and/or onions.

Hawthorn

To improve the circulation of the blood and strengthen the heart muscle, drink tea prepared from the fruit, leaves, or flowers of the hawthorn tree (*Crataegus* spp.).

Red Beets

Eat large quantities of red beets to lower high blood pressure.

Comments

Digitalis or foxglove is a known cardiotonic drug. It acts to increase the force of contraction of the heart muscle, thus causing it to empty more effectively. Because the drug is an extremely potent one, its highly purified constituents known as glycosides are now used in medicine to provide exact doses. Overdoses can be quite harmful, even fatal. Thus, the consumption of a water extract made from inexact quantities of unstandardized leaves as described in the informant's recipe is certainly not to be recommended.

It now appears that certain constituents in hawthorn do have a beneficial effect upon the heart and circulatory system. The tea would therefore act to dilate the blood vessels, especially the coronary vessels, thus reducing the tendency to angina attack. It also apparently has a direct, favorable effect on the heart itself. This action is slow to develop, doing so after repeated use, but toxicity is almost lacking, becoming apparent only in very large doses. Hawthorn is widely used in Europe where it enjoys the reputation of being a useful heart tonic. The wisdom of self-treating any abnormal heart condition is quite another matter. This is probably emphasized by the relative paucity of cures submitted for such conditions.

Consumption of relatively large amounts of raw garlic (about 2 ounces or more weekly) or onions (1.3 pounds weekly) does apparently have a beneficial effect on high blood pressure and the various factors leading to or associated with it. Amounts this large of either herb would seldom be included in a typical American diet.

⧉Colds and Flu⧉

Asafetida

Hang a small bag containing asafetida (*Ferula* spp.) around a child's neck to ward off colds during the winter months.

> *It may have helped as no one wanted to come near the person wearing it.* Irene Lankford

Balm

To relieve a cold and overcome the accompanying fatigue, drink balm tea (*Melissa officinalis*).

Boneset

Boneset herb (*Eupatorium perfoliatum*) is made into a tea useful for colds, croup, and flu.

Boneset, Feverweed, Pennyroyal

Boil boneset (*Eupatorium perfoliatum*), feverweed (*Chrysanthemum parthenium*), and pennyroyal (*Hedeoma pulegioides*) in water until the color turns and drink ½ teacupful, either plain or sweetened, to cure the flu.

> *It's a pill to take, but it'll kill or cure.* Lina Bell Duncan

Bread, Hot Milk

Apply bread soaked in hot milk to relieve swollen neck glands.

Camphor

To ward off chest colds, wrap a piece of gum camphor in a bit of cheesecloth and hang on a string that is long enough for the cloth bag to make contact with the chest when the bag is hung around the neck.

Camphor

Put camphor spirits on a cloth and apply to the chest to cure a cold.

Castor Oil, Turpentine

For chest colds, mix 2 tablespoonfuls of castor oil with 1 tablespoonful of turpentine spirits. Warm and rub on the chest. Cover with a warm cloth.

Catnip

Catnip tea (*Nepeta cataria*) is good for a cold.

Crab Apple

Swollen glands in the neck accompanying a cold can be relieved with a crab apple poultice (*Malus* spp.).

Dittany

Hot dittany tea (*Cunila origanoides*) is an effective cold remedy.

Egg, Milk, Sugar, Nutmeg

To cure a cold, beat together the yolk of an egg, 1 teaspoonful of sugar, and a cup of hot milk. Add the white of an egg beaten to a foam and a little nutmeg. Drink it very hot before going to bed.

Elderberry Flowers

Drink tea made from elderberry flowers (*Sambucus canadensis*) to cure a cold.

Flaxseed

Apply a flaxseed (*Linum usitatissimum*) poultice for chest colds. This is made by boiling the seeds in a little water, mixing with cornmeal, and, after application, covering with a clean cloth.

Flaxseed, Sugar, Honey, Lemon

A good cure for colds is prepared by boiling 2 ounces of flaxseed (*Linum usitatissimum*) in 1 quart of water; strain and add 2 ounces of rock candy, ½ pint of honey, and the juice of 3 lemons. Mix, boil well, cool, and bottle. Drink ½ cupful before meals and 1 cupful at bedtime—the hotter the better.

Food

Feed a cold and starve a fever.

Ginger

To cure a cold, drink strong ginger tea (*Zingiber officinale*) prepared by steeping a teaspoon of ginger in ½ pint of boiling water and adding a tablespoon of sugar. Then jump in bed, cover up completely, head and all, and sweat it out.

Goose Grease

Rub the throat and chest with goose grease to cure a cold.

Goose Grease

To cure colds, rub goose grease on the chest, the palms of the hands, and the soles of the feet.

Goose or Skunk Grease, Camphor or Turpentine

For a cold in the chest, rub the chest and back with goose or skunk grease to which camphor or turpentine has been added. Cover with warm flannel.

Herbal Mixture

To cure a cold, take the following:

   3 handfuls of horehound (*Marrubium vulgare*),
   3 handfuls of spignet (*Aralia racemosa*),
   3 handfuls of comfrey (*Symphytum officinale*), and
   1 handful of Indian turnip (*Arisaema triphyllum*).

Put all in a large pot, add water, and boil it down to 1 quart. Then put in 1 quart of vinegar and boil down to 1 quart. Strain out the plant material and add 1 quart of honey to the clear liquid. Take as needed.

From a receipt book dated 1836—attributed to the father of D. W. Shauman.

Hickory Bark

Make tea from the bark that scales up on a shagbark hickory tree (*Carya ovata*) to cure a cold.

Horehound

Horehound leaves (*Marrubium vulgare*) are dried and made into tea for the common cold. Sweeten and thicken with molasses.

Hot Water

Soak your feet in hot water to cure a cold.

Kerosene, Lard

Mix kerosene and lard, rub on the chest, and cover with a cloth to cure a cold.

Lemon

Drink hot lemonade and take hot foot baths to keep from catching cold.

Lemon

To cure a cold, drink hot lemonade made from the whole lemon—rind and all.

Mullein

Drink mullein leaf tea (*Verbascum thapsus*) to break up a cold.

Mullein Leaves

To cure bronchitis, smoke dried and powdered mullein leaves (*Verbascum thapsus*) in a new clay pipe in which no tobacco has ever been smoked. Draw the smoke well into the throat, swallowing some occasionally. Use this treatment 3 or 4 times daily.

Mullein, Cinnamon, Cloves

For a cold, drink tea made from mullein leaves (*Verbascum thapsus*) with a little cinnamon and cloves added.

Mustard Plaster

A mustard plaster for chest colds or other pains is prepared by mixing equal parts of ground mustard (*Brassica* spp.) and flour with the white of an egg and sufficient water to make a paste. Spread on cloth and apply to the affected parts.

Nutmeg

Apply a nutmeg poultice to the chest to cure the croup or a bad cold.

> *I have used this remedy with good results since 1924.* Beulah Ramey

Nutmeg

A simple and effective remedy for colds or soreness of the chest is to spread lard or vaseline on a piece of knitted underwear, sprinkle liberally with nutmeg, and apply.

> *Used by my great-grandmother in the 1860s.* Jim Whiteford

Onions

To make an onion poultice for chest colds, fry the onions in grease until tender, drain, make into poultice, and apply to chest. Change frequently and keep patient warm. It is a sure way to break up colds. The liquid drained off is sweetened with sugar and given to babies with colds. It also causes them to sleep well.

> *I think all winter long we had grease and onions on the stove.* Dorothy Hoffman

Onions

Eat lots of onions or drink onion juice to cure a cold.

Onions

To clear head-cold congestion in a child, chop and fry 2 medium sized onions until they begin to turn clear. Put them in a cloth several layers thick (an old diaper is good) and pin to the inside of a shirt or gown over the chest area, making certain it is not hot enough to burn. The nasal passages soon will open, and the child can sleep peacefully.

Onions

Hang onions in every room to keep members of the family from catching cold.

Pennyroyal

Pennyroyal tea (*Hedeoma pulegioides*) is good for colds and flu.

Peppermint, Sugar

Drink a few drops of peppermint spirit in a glass of water sweetened with sugar to relieve a cold.

Peppermint; Spearmint

Drink peppermint (*Mentha piperita*) or spearmint (*Mentha spicata*) tea to cure a cold.

Queen-of-the-Meadow; Boneset

Both queen-of-the-meadow (*Eupatorium purpureum*) and boneset (*Eupatorium perfoliatum*) are made into teas that are highly valued treatments for colds and flu.

Quinine

To ward off a chill and avoid catching cold, take a capsule of quinine.

Red Beets

Eat raw, ground, red beets to cure a cold that has settled in the lungs.

Sage

To break up a cold, drink sage tea prepared by placing a large pinch of dry sage (*Salvia officinalis*) in a heavy crockery cup (never use metal). Fill with boiling water, cover with a saucer, and let steep for 5 minutes. Strain, sweeten a bit, and drink while still hot just before bedtime. Do this for several nights and you will be relieved of your cold.

An old German recipe. Alice Whiteford

Salt Water

Head colds are eased by sniffing warm salt water up the nose.

Sedge Grass

Sedge grass root (*Carex* spp.) is boiled in water to make a drink that is good for colds and fever.

Sheep Sorrel (Yellow Wood Sorrel)

To prevent colds, take a teacupful of yellow-flowered sorrel (*Oxalis stricta*), an ounce of sugar, a dash of nutmeg, and a pint of boiling water. Steep in a teapot for at least 3 minutes before drinking.

Skunk Grease

Skunk grease is recommended for swollen glands in the neck.

Soot, Pine Tar, Camphor, Turpentine, Tallow, Lard

Mix mutton tallow, lard, soot, pine tar, camphor, and turpentine and apply to the chest as a poultice to break up congestion.

> *It will also fumigate your house and rid it of rats, mice, wasps, bedbugs, and roaches.* Bill Thomas

Summer Savory

Take tea made from summer savory (*Satureja hortensis*) to cure a cold.

Thyme

Thyme tea (*Thymus vulgaris*) will relieve the symptoms of a cold.

Tobacco Dregs

To clear up nasal congestion, light the dregs in the bottom of a pipe and blow the smoke at the person, who should breathe very deeply of it.

Turpentine, Lard

Mix turpentine oil with lard and rub on the chest to cure the congestion associated with a cold.

Turpentine, Lard

Heat turpentine oil and lard together in a saucer, rub on the chest and keep covered with a warm wool cloth.

Vinegar

To clear up sinus trouble associated with a cold, inhale the fumes of vinegar. First heat a brick very hot in the fireplace. Make a little tent over the brick with a thick blanket or comforter, stick your head under it, and inhale the vapor formed when the vinegar is dropped slowly on the brick. Then take the comforter, wrap yourself up in it, and after you have perspired freely, go to sleep. When you wake up, your sinus trouble will be over.

Whiskey

A certain remedy for colds and influenza is to hang your hat on the bedpost and drink whiskey until you see two hats.

Whiskey, Lemon, Sugar

For a cold, drink whiskey warmed with lemon juice and sugar.

Wild Mint

The symptoms of a cold are relieved with tea made from wild mint. (*Blephilia, Pycnanthemum,* or *Monarda* spp.).

Wild Onions

To treat nasal irritation and congestion associated with a cold, chop up the bulbs of several wild onions (*Allium cepa*) and drop into a saucepan containing a small amount of boiling water. Let boil for 5 minutes. Remove from heat, cover container and your head with a towel, and inhale the vapor.

Wild Strawberry Leaves

Take tea made from wild strawberry leaves (*Fragaria virginiana*) to cure a cold.

Yarrow

Yarrow tea (*Achillea millefolium*) is good for colds.

Comments

There is really very little one can do to overcome the viral infections causing colds and flu except to alleviate the unpleasant symptoms as much as possible and make the patient more comfortable. Since the condition often involves loss of fluid (dehydration), all of the various teas ranging, alphabetically, from balm to yarrow are useful in keeping the body well supplied with liquid. They consist primarily of water, which is itself an effective expectorant, stimulating the secretions of the bronchial mucosa. Water vapor (steam) also has a soothing demulcent effect.

In addition, some of the herbs themselves, such as horehound, act as expectorants and further stimulate the helpful secretions. Others, such as mullein, also contain mucilaginous constituents which soothe the irritated mucous membranes. Still others—peppermint, ginger, thyme, etc.—possess aromatic and antiseptic properties which tend to relieve congestion.

The penetrating nature of the aroma of onions apparently accounts for the highly popular use of onion poultices applied to break up chest colds and relieve congestion. However, it is also recommended that they be eaten raw as a treatment or even hung up in bunches around the house to prevent the inhabitants from catching cold in the first place. Hoosiers will be interested in the recent reports in European newspapers that Queen Elizabeth II takes freshly pressed onion juice to relieve her head colds. At least we are in good company in attributing great efficacy to this popular herb. Its widespread use makes one wonder if there is not more to it than is currently believed by practitioners of conventional medicine.

Aromatic materials such as camphor, kerosene, turpentine oil, vinegar, and skunk grease are probably most useful for their penetrating properties in providing some relief from nasal congestion. The mustard plaster stimulates circulation in the area to which it is applied (often the chest) and brings a feeling of relief. Poultices from flaxseed or crab apples will at least keep the area to which they are applied warm and moist. Whiskey will not cure a cold, but if the sufferer drinks enough, especially enough to see double as one informant recommended, he will certainly forget about the cold for a while. Hot lemonade is useful not only for the liquid it supplies but for its vitamin C content as well. It will also act to decrease congestion, as will any hot drink.

The offensive odor of the resinous material asafetida, sometimes known as devils' dung, has no power to ward off colds per se, but as one correspondent pointed out, it does tend to keep people with colds (and those without) away from a person who wears a bagful of it hung around the neck. Probably the same reasoning applies to a bag of camphor worn in a similar manner.

⇒Cold Sores⇐

Cornmeal

Apply a cornmeal poultice to cure a fever blister (cold sore).

Ear Wax

To heal a cold sore quickly, put ear wax on it.

Comments

Cold sores, or fever blisters as they are sometimes called, are caused by the herpes simplex virus. The suggested treatments would, at best, be modestly palliative in nature.

⇒Constipation⇐

Butternut

To relieve constipation, collect the root or stem bark of the butternut tree (*Juglans cinerea*), place in water, and boil down until the liquid becomes quite thick. This is made into pills that have a mild laxative effect.

Castor Oil

Use castor oil as a laxative.

Elderberries

The juice of fresh elderberries (*Sambucus canadensis*) is a quick and mild purgative.

Epsom Salts

Epsom salts dissolved in water is an efficient laxative.

Hot Water

A pleasant alternative to the customary doses of castor oil or epsom salts is simply to drink a cup of plain hot water, instead of coffee, for breakfast every morning.

>*Very effective!* Dorris B. Layman

Mayapple

Drink tea made from mayapple roots (*Podophyllum peltatum*) to relieve constipation. Alternatively, take about ¼ teaspoonful of the powdered root.

Peach Tree Bark

Drink tea made from peach tree bark (*Prunus persica*) to overcome constipation.

Slippery Elm Bark

Chew the inner bark of the slippery elm tree (*Ulmus fulva*) to cure constipation.

Slippery Elm Bark

Slippery elm bark may also be made into a tea that is drunk to relieve constipation.

Violet Petals

A syrup of violet petals (*Viola* spp.) relieves constipation in children.

Wild Senna

Tea made from wild senna leaves (*Cassia hebecarpa*) is an excellent purge for the system.

Comments

Laxatives play a significant role in folk medicine, and it was somewhat surprising that a greater number of them were not supplied by the informants. Possibly the old standbys, castor oil and epsom salts, are so widely known, so readily available, and efficient, that it was unnecessary to seek out additional remedies. Some are, however, listed under other headings. The neuritis cure composed of figs, raisins, senna, slippery elm, and the like is an excellent example.

Of the products listed, the one which should be used with greatest caution, if at all, is mayapple. The root is a drastic purgative, and much more suitable products to relieve constipation are readily available.

⇗Contagious Diseases⇖ (Prevention of)

Asafetida

Put a lump of asafetida (*Ferula* spp.) in a cloth bag and hang it around the neck to ward off measles, whooping cough, mumps, and all other contagious diseases.

> *I used this on myself and my children and it really works.* Maude Nellis

> *But I do remember Aunt Vonda Mae got the whooping cough while she was wearing one.* Ethel Ellett

Onions

Slice up onions and place them in saucers around the house to ward off contagious disease germs, especially diphtheria.

Comments

The use of both these products to ward off disease has been discussed in the section Colds and Flu. The same comments apply here. The statements of two of the informants quoted under asafetida are revealing.

⇴Coughs and Croup⇷

Alum, Egg White

For croup, add a piece of alum to the white of an egg and stir until it becomes liquid. Then drink it.

Alum, Molasses

To relieve the croup, administer a mixture of alum and molasses.

Balm of Gilead, Honey, Lemon

Put a handful of fresh buds in 1 quart of water and slowly simmer down to 1 pint before straining. Add 1 pound of honey and the juice of 3 lemons. Take in teaspoonful doses to relieve cough.

> *Balm of gilead buds* (Populus candicans) *were used to prepare cough medicine in Miami County, Indiana, about 1888.* Florence Field

Butter, Sugar

For coughs in children, administer sugar mixed with ½ teaspoonful of butter.

Flaxseed

Drink boiled flaxseed tea (*Linum usitatissimum*) for coughs and sore throats.

Flaxseed, Sodium Citrate, Glycerin, Lemon, Peppermint

Foolproof cough medicine: Put 1 tablespoonful of whole flaxseed (*Linùm usitatissimum*) in a pint of water and boil for 20 to 30 minutes. Strain out the seeds and add 1 ounce of sodium citrate, 2 tablespoonfuls of glycerin, the juice of a lemon, and 2 or 3 drops of peppermint essence. Take a table-spoonful every hour or two for 1 or 2 days as needed.

Garlic, Vinegar, Honey, (Whiskey)

Garlic cough syrup: Take 1 or more fresh, large bulbs of garlic and cook until soft in 1 cup of apple cider vinegar. Add ½ cup of honey (or 1 cup of sugar) and simmer to make a syrup. Use as is for coughs or after mixing half and half with whiskey. The half-and-half mixture may be put in small fruit jars and sealed for use during the winter.

> *The garlic cough syrup fixed this way does not taste bad. One of my grandkids would pretend she had a cough the minute she came in the house, so I would give her some. That is why it can be fixed without the whiskey. Try it, you'll like it.* Margie M. Fogleman

Honey

A teaspoonful of honey will quiet a cough.

Honey, Salt

Croup is treated with a mixture comprised of 1 teaspoonful of honey and 1 of salt.

Honey, Vinegar, Glycerin

An effective homemade cough syrup is prepared by mixing 1 cup of honey, ½ cup of cider vinegar, and 2 tablespoonfuls of glycerin. Stir before using. Take 1 teaspoonful at bedtime or as needed.

> *This will stop a cough when all others fail.*
> N. Davidson

Honey, Vinegar; (Olive Oil)

Honey mixed with vinegar is an effective cough treatment. A little sweet oil (olive oil) may also be added to the mixture.

Horehound, Sugar

Boil horehound (*Marrubium vulgare*) leaves in water and add sugar to make an effective cough syrup.

Horehound, Sugar, Menthol

Boil a handful of horehound leaves (*Marrubium vulgare*) in a quart of water and let stand for 2 hours. Add 2 cups of brown sugar and boil for ½ hour. Then take a good pinch of menthol crystals and let them dissolve in the syrup. Take 2 teaspoonfuls as needed.

Hot Water

For a tight, hoarse, dry cough, just frequently sip hot water—as hot as can be borne. It will give immediate and lasting relief.

Lemon, Sugar

Lemon cough syrup: Boil 3 fresh lemons until soft and slice them on a pound of brown sugar. Stew together for 15 to 20 minutes to form a rich syrup. Cool. Add 1 tablespoonful of sweet almond oil. Take 1 or more spoonfuls for troublesome cough.

Licorice Root, Rock Candy, Honey

Boil licorice root (*Glycyrrhiza glabra*) in water and add rock candy and honey to make a thick syrup. Take 1 tablespoonful for cough.

Mosses

To cure a cough, make and drink a strong tea from equal parts of the loose, coarse moss growing on white oak (*Quercus alba*), white maple (*Acer saccharinum*), and white ash (*Fraxinus americana*) trees.

Mullein, Honey

Mullein cough syrup: In the fall, about October, when the sap of the mullein plants (*Verbascum thapsus*) has run down to the roots and the stalk is brown, dig up 3 or 4 roots and cut off the stalks. Scrub the roots thoroughly with a vegetable brush and water. Place in a large pot, cover with water, and let it steam, not boil, over a slow fire all day. Turn off the heat and let steep overnight. Repeat the cooking and soaking process the second day and night. On the third morning, remove the roots and strain the liquid through cheesecloth. Sweeten to taste with honey, sorghum, or sugar. Pour into pint jars or bottles and seal. Take by the spoonful for coughs.

> *This recipe was used by my mother, grand-mother, and great-grandmother. It is the only cough remedy taken by me and by my seven brothers and sisters for many years.* Stella Vanderhoef

Onion

Give onion tea for the croup.

Onion

For croup, cook a slice of onion in a saucer and give the juice to the child.

From my grandmother, a full-blooded Indian.
Mrs. Leslie Peters

Onions, Sugar

For croup in children, bake onions, chop, and squeeze through gauze. Add a small amount of granulated sugar to the squeezings. Give as needed.

Onions, Sugar

A variation of the above treatment for croup is to cut an onion into thin slices and cover each slice completely with brown sugar. Let it dissolve and collect the syrup thus formed. Use as needed.

Onion, Sugar

Make onion cough syrup by cutting 3 good-sized onions up fine and adding a large amount of sugar. Set it on the stove on low heat and let it make its own syrup. Strain the mixture. Give 1 teaspoonful every hour.

Onion, Sugar

A similar onion cough syrup is made by first frying the onions in grease which is then poured off into another pan. To this, add brown sugar, a little water, and cook until thick. The dose is 1 teaspoonful every ½ hour.

Rock Candy

To relieve coughs, suck on rock candy.

Rock Candy, Brandy (Whiskey)

Dissolve ¼ cup of rock candy in 1 cup of brandy or whiskey. Take a tablespoonful for severe and persistent coughs.

Rosin, Alum, Ginger, Pepper, Butter, Honey

For a cough, mix 2 tablespoonfuls of rosin, 2 of alum, 2 of ginger, and 2 of black pepper with 2 of fresh butter and a saucer of honey. Simmer together. Take 1 teaspoonful at bedtime.

Skunk Cabbage, Vinegar, Honey

Make a cough syrup by simmering down 4 ounces of skunk cabbage root (*Symplocarpus foetidus*) in a quart of vinegar to about 1½ pints. Strain, add 1 pint of honey, simmer, and skim to clear. Take 6 or 7 teaspoonfuls per day.

Skunk Oil

At the very first sign of croup, skunk oil (grease) is rubbed on the chest and covered with a flannel cloth.

> *My mother got a bottle of skunk oil every winter for twenty-five cents from an old trapper. It was light yellow and had the consistency of cold cream. It was a sure cure.* Lucile M. Imes

Swamp Alder

Make tea for a cough from the small branches or bark of the swamp alder (*Alnus* spp.).

Tobacco

For croup, spread lard on a cloth and cover either with snuff or with tobacco taken from a cigaret. Put the cloth on the chest and cover with another warm cloth to drive it in.

Turpentine or Kerosene, Sugar

To treat a cough take a spoonful of turpentine spirits or kerosene mixed with sugar.

Turpentine, Pepper, Sugar

For coughs, take a pinch of a mixture of sugar and pepper, moistened with turpentine spirits.

Violet Petals, Sugar

A syrup made of violet petals (*Viola* spp.) is excellent for coughs and sore throats in children.

Wheat Plant

Tea made from the green wheat plant (*Triticum aestivum*) is good for the croup.

Wild Ginger, Sugar

Boil wild ginger root (*Asarum* spp.) in water, strain, and add sufficient sugar to make a thick syrup. This is given in teaspoonful doses to relieve coughs.

Comments

Coughing is really a useful mechanism enabling a person to clear obstructions from the throat. Unfortunately, in the case of some types of upper respiratory infections in which large quantities of phlegm and mucus accumulate, the desire to cough becomes so nagging and the act itself so persistent and severe that measures to alleviate it become necessary. These are ordinarily of two types. The first involves some compound such as codeine, which acts directly on the brain to depress that part of it responsible for the cough mechanism.

The second involves palliative treatment of the throat itself so that the cough mechanism is not triggered. All of the remedies in this listing are of the second type.

Palliative treatment includes the use of expectorants that stimulate the secretions of the bronchial mucosa, of demulcents that soothe and provide a protective coating for the throat, and of astringents that exert a drawing or puckering effect on the tissue. Some products or recipes combine all of these properties.

Horehound, a favorite cough remedy, is an effective expectorant due to its bitter principle marrubiin. Because of its viscous, adhesive nature, honey is a typical demulcent as are mullein leaves due to their content of mucilage. Alum is a typical astringent, but many volatile oils (e.g., turpentine oil) also possess astringent properties. Licorice is both an expectorant and a demulcent.

Again onions seem to occupy the most prominent position in terms of cough preparations. A garlic cough syrup with added vinegar, honey, and sometimes whiskey, is also highly recommended. One correspondent was kind enough to send me a sample of the mullein root and honey syrup, so I can personally vouch for its effectiveness.

✥Cure-Alls✥

Chicken Soup

Eat chicken soup to cure anything.

> *The oldest Jewish cure for anything. My mother, grandmothers, great-grandmothers, etc., all swear by it.* Sue Henderson

Milkweed Root

Dried powdered milkweed or silkweed root (*Asclepias syriaca*) is given for nervous disorders, dropsy (as a diuretic), high fevers, as a blood purifier, nerve strengthener, laxative, and to cure the piles. In larger doses, up to 1 teaspoonful, it is good for snake or spider bites. Mix with a little honey to make it easier to take.

Rest

Rest.

> *It is really the best cure for everything!* Julia Koch LaSelle

Comments

Certainly no one would dispute the merits of chicken soup and rest as useful therapeutic measures for almost any ailment. The use of milkweed root as a panacea is more controversial. Although the information regarding its use as a Hoosier remedy dates back nearly 150 years, we really know little more about it today than did the Indiana pioneers of that era. Further scientific and medicinal studies of milkweed and many other herbal remedies are certainly needed.

⇨Cuts, Bruises, and Abrasions⇦

Castor Oil

Rub castor oil on bruises to make them disappear quickly.

Cow Manure

Fresh cow manure is applied to cuts on the feet to hasten healing.

Kerosene

Kerosene applied to a cut will help it heal.

Knot Grass

Apply the juice from knot grass (*Polygonum aviculare*) to bruised areas. Repeat this 3 times a day and especially at bedtime to obtain relief.

Peach Tree Leaves

For a stone bruise, mash peach tree leaves (*Prunus persica*) in sweet cream and apply.

Plantain

Bind a green plantain leaf (*Plantago* spp.) to a severe bruise or abrasion.

> *My whole growing up years were spent with a plantain leaf bound to my knees! I fell down a lot. That plant actually draws out infection.* Betty Kingston—the girl with the green knees

Red Pepper

Apply red pepper directly to heal a cut.

Rosin, Turpentine, (Camphor)

A useful salve for healing cuts is prepared as follows:

Rosin	lump the size of a hickory nut
Beeswax	lump the size of a walnut
Tallow	lump the size of a goose egg

Melt together and add 2 tablespoonfuls of turpentine oil. Add a little camphor gum, if desired. Apply as necessary.

Starch; Butter

To keep a bruise from discoloring, either apply a little corn starch or arrowroot starch that has been moistened with cold water or rub the spot with common table butter.

Tobacco

A moist cud of tobacco is useful for healing cuts. Simply apply to the affected area and wrap it with a cloth.

Turpentine

Apply turpentine oil to help heal minor cuts.

Veal, Lettuce

To reduce the swelling of a bruised (black) eye, apply a thin strip of very cold veal, cover with a lettuce leaf, and then bandage. Repeat several times as the meat becomes warm.

Yarrow

Treat minor cuts and bruises with a salve made from the yarrow plant (*Achillea millefolium*).

Comments

Since minor injuries of this sort normally heal rather well without treatment of any kind, the remedies supplied by Indiana informants seem mostly innocuous, if not superfluous. Some, such as turpentine oil, red pepper, and even kerosene, no doubt possess styptic or antiseptic properties. Others, such as cow manure and chewed tobacco, may likely prove more harmful than helpful.

Two of the remedies are of special interest. The application of plantain leaves to bruises and abrasions as well as blisters, wounds, bee stings, and even sore eyes was frequently recommended by informants. The same information has come to my attention from European sources where the leaves are also applied locally to such affected areas with reported successful results. Yet scientists know little, if anything, about the constituents of plantain leaves that might be reponsible for promoting healing and preventing infection in injuries of this type.

The same may be said for peach tree leaves which are also reported useful as local applications on bruises and wounds, and with less success, to treat boils. The cause of their purported effectiveness in such situations remains obscure.

It is quite rational to apply something cold to a bruised eye to prevent discoloration because the cold constricts the ruptured capillaries and tends to prevent the blood from seeping out of them and becoming dark. However, it is no longer rational to use a costly meat like veal for this purpose, and the lettuce leaf simply acts to help contain the moisture. Applications of ice or very cold water would probably be equally effective and much less expensive.

⇒Deafness⇐

Turtle Oil

Boil the oil from a turtle, cool, and drop it in the ear(s) to cure deafness.

Comments

This remedy may belong more in the category of magic and myth than in the realm of reality. As such, it probably should not be included in this listing. Still, because it was the only reported cure for deafness, we have decided to include it.

⤳Diabetes⤲

Grapefruit

For diabetes, wash and grind 6 white grapefruits. Add 6 quarts of water and mix well. Drink 1 quart of the juice daily.

Alum, Milk

Dissolve a pinch of alum in ½ glass of milk and drink 3 times a day.

Comments

A large number of herbs have been reported by various peoples around the world as being effective in the treatment of diabetes. It was rather surprising, therefore, that only these two nonherbal remedies were reported by Hoosier correspondents. Neither is of any value in treating the disease.

⇒Diaphoretics⇐ (to Induce Perspiration)

Burdock Seed

To cause sweating, take ½ teaspoonful of pulverized burdock seed (*Arctium minus*) in a little warm water.

Comments

Sweating was long considered as an important method of ridding the body of toxic wastes. Consequently, diaphoretics or agents to induce sweating were once very widely used in medicine, as were emetics to promote vomiting, laxatives and cathartics to expel solid waste, and, of course, blood letting to remove "bad" blood. These methods, with the possible exception of laxatives and cathartics, have fallen by the wayside and are seldom used today. Only a single, specific diaphoretic herb was reported by informants, but it should be noted that causing perspiration is still an important part of such remedies as the vinegar inhalation treatment for colds described in the section Colds and Flu and the various recipes noted in the two sections Fevers and Malaria.

⇒Diarrhea and Dysentery⇐

Alum Root

Take alum root tea (*Heuchera americana*) for diarrhea.

Blackberry Roots

Wash and cut blackberry roots (*Rubus* spp.) into small pieces. Add boiling water and steep until a strong tea is made. Strain and add sugar sufficient to make a syrup. Bottle, cork, and seal. Take a teaspoonful every 1 to 3 hours for diarrhea.

Blackberries

A balsam made by boiling wild blackberries (*Rubus* spp.) in water and straining the resulting liquid is an excellent remedy for dysentery.

> *My grandmother got this from the Indians.*
> Lillian N. Rosner

Blackberries

To cure diarrhea in the summertime (summer flux), simply eat blackberries (*Rubus* spp.). Blackberry wine is also effective.

Buckhorn Plantain

For diarrhea, make a tea from the dried seed spikes of buckhorn or English plantain (*Plantago lanceolata*). (Original recipe from Charles Elmer Fox)

> *Using this, I cured myself of a three-year bout*
> *of recurring diarrhea.* Sylvia Schwartz

Chicken Gizzard

To cure chronic diarrhea in an infant, cut the lining from a chicken gizzard and dry it. Then put it in boiling water to make a tea. Give 1 teaspoonful to the baby every ½ hour.

Corn

Eat parched corn to cure diarrhea.

Dogfennel

Drink tea made from the yellow middle part of dogfennel flowers (*Anthemis cotula*) to cure diarrhea.

Dogwood

Tea made from the bark of the dogwood tree (*Cornus florida*) will cure diarrhea.

Flour, Sugar, Salt, Nutmeg

For diarrhea, brown dry wheat flour in a tin pan. Then put the flour in a bowl and pour a little boiling water into it, stirring until the mixture is the consistency of gravy. Add sugar, salt, and nutmeg. Take 1 teaspoonful every ½ hour.

Grapes

Eat grapes with the skins on to prevent diarrhea.

Mare's Milk

Drink mare's milk to cure the flux (diarrhea).

Mare's Tail

Take 20 leaves, green or dry, of *Erigeron canadense*, commonly known as horse weed or mare's tail, add 1 quart of boiling water, and steep to make a tea. Add sugar to taste. For diarrhea, drink 4 ounces first, then 2 ounces every 2 hours until cured.

> *It will work better than anything I know of.*
> Philip R. LeGrand

Nutmeg

Drink nutmeg tea for diarrhea.

Orange Peel

Chronic diarrhea can be cured by drinking freely of tea made from orange peels and sweetened with sugar. Use for 24 to 36 hours as necessary.

Ragweed

To cure diarrhea, select only the top leaves of ragweed plants (*Ambrosia elatior*), wash carefully, take a large pinch of them, and chew. Swallow the juices produced during the chewing process, but spit out the leaves themselves.

Rhubarb, Baking Soda, Peppermint

For diarrhea, take 1 teaspoonful of powdered rhubarb root (*Rheum rhaponticum*), 1 teaspoonful of baking soda, and add 1 teacup of boiling water plus 1 or 2 drops of peppermint oil. Take 1 tablespoonful 3 times a day.

Rhubarb, Wild Cherry

To make a syrup for treating dysentery, take a handful each of rhubarb root (*Rheum rhaponticum*) and wild cherry bark (*Prunus serotina*). Add water, 4 tablespoonfuls of sugar, simmer a while, and add a little brandy. Take 1 tablespoonful every 15 minutes as long as necessary.

Smartweed

Boil the smartweed plant (*Polygonum punctatum*) in water and drink the beverage to control diarrhea.

Smartweed

Smartweed tea (*Polygonum punctatum*) will remedy diarrhea.

Spotted Spurge

Drink iced tea made from fluxweed (*Euphorbia supina*), also known as prostrate spurge, spotted spurge, or milk purslane, for diarrhea. It is also effective for intestinal flu.

> *A friend showed me the herb and it worked like a charm for bowel trouble. I have used it over the years on children, grandchildren, and tiny babies. In fact, I have a pot of it on my stove right now and am drinking it myself. I am eighty-seven years old. We have some drying for next winter. A friend—a trained nurse— used it successfully for chronic colitis.* Mrs. Charles Newman

Sweet Life Everlasting

Sweet life everlasting herb (*Gnaphalium obtusifolium*) is made into a tea that is a very useful remedy for diarrhea and dysentery.

> *I knew of a case where a person who was suffering with flux and had been given up by the attending physician was cured by drinking copious draughts of milk in which this herb had been boiled.* Charles C. Deam

Comments

Treatments for diarrhea and dysentery function basically in two ways. They either exert an astringent or puckering effect on the intestinal tract or they act as demulcents to coat and protect the irritated lining of the bowel. Some products combine both of these types of treatment.

Alum root, blackberries, and rhubarb, for example, are primarily astringents. Incidentally, the rhubarb root referred to in these recipes is that of the common garden rhubarb (*Rheum rhaponticum*) which is rich in astringent tannins. It is not the so-called Indian rhubarb (*Rheum emodi, Rheum webbianum,* etc.) which is often sold by dealers in herbs and which contains anthraquinones. These cause Indian rhubarb root to have exactly the opposite effect of garden rhubarb root, acting as a laxative instead of helping cure diarrhea.

The parched corn and mare's milk (cow's milk is also modestly effective) act primarily as protective demulcents. The combinations of flour and nutmeg or rhubarb and baking soda provide both astringent and the protective effects. Probably all of the recipes listed are more or less effective treatments for simple diarrhea.

➬Drunkenness ➬

Honey

Administer large amounts of honey—6 teaspoonfuls every 20 minutes until a total of 2 pounds is given—to cure drunkenness. This treatment will also abolish the desire to drink liquor.

Comments

The main contituents of honey are dextrose and fructose. There is no reason to believe that administration of either honey or these simple sugars in large amounts would cause an intoxicated person to sober up more quickly or would reduce the craving for alcohol.

⋙Earache⋘

Chewing Tobacco

Insert a moist wad of chewing tobacco into the ear to relieve earache.

Hops

Treat earache by applying small muslin bags of warm, but not wet, hops (*Humulus lupulus*). Tie them over the ears at night with a large kerchief.

Olive Oil

Put a few drops of warm sweet oil (olive oil) directly into the ear to cure an earache. Then plug the ear with cotton.

Onion

Drop juice from a roasted onion into the ear to cure an earache.

Onion, Tobacco

An earache is treated by roasting together a mixture of onion and tobacco. Squeeze a drop of the juice from them into the ear.

Pepper, Olive Oil

For earache, take a small piece of absorbent cotton, make a depression in the center, and fill with powdered black pepper. Make into a ball with the pepper in the center and tie it up with a thread. Dip it in olive oil and insert into the ear. It will give instant relief.

Salt

Cloth bags of salt are heated and held to the ear as a compress to cure an earache.

Salt Pork

To relieve an earache, cut a piece of salt pork into a pointed strip and insert in the ear.

Tobacco Smoke

To cure an earache, blow warm tobacco smoke gently into the ear.

> *I loved this and often developed an earache.*
> Madge Ellett

Urine

Pour warm urine in the ear to cure an earache.

Urine

Put a few drops of urine from a person of the opposite sex in the ear to cure earache.

Comments

Most of the treatments for earache seem to depend on applying warmth in some way to the painful area. Blowing tobacco smoke in the ear, a very popular treatment reported by eight informants, would, however, provide only a transient change in temperature at best. Consequently, one wonders if the nicotine or tar or some other ingredient in the smoke does not provide an additional effect.

Dropping in warm olive oil has long been a standard method of relieving earache; presumably warm urine functions in the same, but somewhat less sanitary, manner. The requirement that the urine be provided by a person of the opposite sex is merely a superstition.

The ubiquitous onion makes its appearance here once again, this time in the form of juice squeezed into the ear from the roasted bulb, either plain or in combination with tobacco. Tobacco by itself was also recommended by several informants in the form of a chewed quid inserted into the ear. All of the liquid preparations mentioned, especially olive oil, would be helpful in softening any impacted ear wax.

⋙Emetics⋘
(to Induce Vomiting)

Lobelia

Pulverized lobelia seeds (*Lobelia inflata*) are the most efficient emetic. The leaves and pods may also be used, but they are less active. Give ½ to 1 teaspoonful together with ½ teaspoonful of red pepper in a little warm water every 15 minutes until vomiting occurs.

Black Mustard

To cause vomiting, give a teaspoonful of whole black mustard seed (*Brassica nigra, B. juncea*). In severe cases, give a tablespoonful.

White Mustard

To induce vomiting, give 1 or 2 teaspoonfuls of pulverized mustard seed (*Brassica alba*) in a little warm water.

Comments

As noted in the section on Diaphoretics, emetics were also once widely used in the treatment of disease. They were thought to be especially effective to remove accumulations of mucus in bronchial complaints. But the herbal practitioner Samuel Thomson and his disciples used the emetic properties of lobelia as a cure for practically every disease.

Now the use of such herbs is restricted primarily to emptying the stomach in cases of poisoning. Even then, lobelia should be used with great caution, if at all, and certainly not in the large doses recommended by the informant; the plant is very toxic. The use of mustard seed is not only safer, but it is also an effective emetic.

⇖Eye Problems⇗

Bread, Milk

For a sore eye, soak a slice of bread in a little milk and tie it over the eye with an old stocking at bedtime. The next morning all of the inflammation will be gone.

Chickweed

Soak chickweed plant (*Stellaria media*) in warm water to prepare a solution that relieves itching and inflammation of the eyes.

Flaxseed

Remove a foreign object from the eye by carefully inserting a moistened whole flaxseed. Close the eye for a few moments and remove the seed. The foreign object will adhere to it.

Flaxseed

For dirt in the eye, carefully place one or two flaxseeds under the eyelid and close for a moment. All of the foreign matter will adhere to the seeds which will gradually work their way out.

Plantain

To relieve soreness of the eyes, apply fresh green plantain leaves (*Plantago* spp.) to the eyelids.

Potato

To cure inflammation of the eyes, a poultice made of raw scraped potato is placed directly on the lids. Thin slices of raw potato may also be used.

Rotten Apple

Soreness of the eye is relieved by applying a rotten apple over it.

Slippery Elm Bark

To treat inflammed eyes, cut some inner bark of the slippery elm (*Ulmus fulva*) into small pieces and soak in warm water until the water becomes mucilaginous. Carefully strain out all the pieces of bark and pat the liquid on the eyelids, allowing some of it to seep into the eyes. It is very soothing.

> *Original recipe from my grandmother who had a smattering of Indian blood and knew many "natural" remedies.* Helen Patrick

Comments

The remedies recommended for application to sore eyes are primarily of a soothing mucilaginous nature and are typified by the bread and milk poultice and the slippery elm bark mucilage. Plantain leaves, on the other hand, are thought to be antiseptic and to confer other beneficial effects.

Placing a moistened flaxseed in the eye for a few moments to remove a foreign object does indeed work. Two different versions of the procedure for using it were submitted by five different correspondents. The flaxseed is rapidly enveloped in a layer of mucilage to which the foreign body—dirt, dust, whatever—will adhere when the seed itself is removed. However, unless the flaxseed is carefully inserted and withdrawn, it may cause considerable irritation on its own. This practice, therefore, like that of placing any nonsterile liquid or substance in the eye, is not recommended.

⇨Falling Hair⇦

Bone Marrow

Falling hair can be stopped by rubbing the head with bone marrow.

Lobelia

Fill a bottle with pulverized lobelia herb (*Lobelia inflata*). Then pour in a mixture of equal parts of brandy or whiskey and olive oil until the bottle is full. Let stand a few days, then bathe the head once a day with the liquid. It will prevent hair loss and restore it after it has fallen out.

Comments

Followers of the Lobelia Doctor, Samuel Thomson, believed the plant could do almost anything in the way of restoring the disordered human body to normal. One of its supposed virtues apparently included the ability to grow hair. Unfortunately, it does not work; neither does the bone marrow treatment. The fat in the latter will serve to keep whatever hair you have neatly in place. It does not smell as nice as some of the "store-bought" hair lotions.

⇗Felons⇖

Beet Leaves, Turpentine, etc.

Apply to a felon a poultice made from 1 teaspoonful each of scorched salt, cornmeal, scraped hard soap, and mashed beet leaves. Add 12 drops of turpentine oil and the yolk of 1 egg. Mix thoroughly.

Egg Shell Membrane

When a felon first appears, wrap it with the inside skin (membrane) from the shell of an egg. When the pressure becomes painful, wet it. Leave it on for 12 hours.

Fleur-de-lis

Apply a poultice of mashed fleur-de-lis root (*Iris* spp.) to cure a felon.

Lemon

A felon on the finger is cured by thrusting the finger into a lemon and keeping it there until the lemon becomes warm. Repeat until 6 lemons have been used.

Onion, Salt

To cure a felon, bake a large onion and mix the soft inner pulp with 2 heaping teaspoonfuls of table salt. Apply twice daily as a poultice.

Comments

Felons are deep, generally pus-producing inflammations of the fingers or toes that usually occur near the ends or around the nails. Folk treatments of them seem to be based on the application of moist materials with potential antiseptic properties.

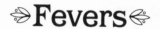# Fevers

Feverfew

To reduce a fever, drink tea made from feverfew (*Chrysanthemum parthenium*).

Ginger

Drink hot ginger tea to break a high fever.

Lemon, Cream of Tartar

An excellent fever drink is made from the juice of lemon, 1 teaspoonful of cream of tartar, and 1 pint of water, sweetened to taste with sugar. Let the patient drink freely of this when thirsty.

Used by my grandmother in the 1860s, the recipe originally came from Germany. Alice Whiteford

Lemon (Orange), Egg White

For fevers, beat the white of 1 egg, add either the juice of 1 lemon or 1 orange, add sugar to taste, and fill the glass with cold water. Drink as necessary.

Marihuana

Dried, crushed marihuana leaves (*Cannabis sativa*) are made into a tea that is very effective in reducing fevers.

Much more effective than aspirin. Anonymous

Onions

Apply onion slices to the bottoms of the feet to "draw off" the heat of a high fever.

Potatoes

Put slices of raw potato in a cloth on the forehead to draw out a fever.

Spicebush

Drink spicebush tea (*Benzoin aestivale*) to cool a fever.

Starve

Feed a cold and starve a fever.

Wild Strawberries

Eat the fruit of the wild strawberry (*Fragaria virginiana*) to reduce fever.

Comments

Perspiring freely is one of the surest ways to reduce a fever. Consequently, most of these remedies involve drinking quantities of hot herb teas which would cause the consumer to sweat. Slices of potato applied to the forehead would have the same beneficial cooling effect as a damp cloth. The other remedies, such as marihuana, onions applied to the soles of the feet, and eating wild strawberries, appear less rational.

⇨Fish Attractant⇦

Sweet Anise; Sweet Cicely

Crush the leaves of sweet anise (*Osmorhiza longistylis*) or sweet cicely (*O. claytoni*) and rub on fishing worms to enhance their flavor and ensure a good catch.

Comments

Fish are known to be attracted by certain odors. One of our informants attributed that effect to the pleasant smelling volatile oils contained in the leaves of these two closely related plants.

✥Fits✥

Cow Parsnip, Pennyroyal

To cure epileptic fits, take a pinch of pulverized cow parsnip (*Heracleum lanatum*) 2 or 3 times daily in pennyroyal (*Hedeoma pulegioides*) tea.

Goldenseal Leaves

The juice of fresh goldenseal leaves (*Hydrastis canadensis*) is a good treatment for fits. Take ½ cupful 2 or 3 times a day.

Sage, Sugar

To prevent fits, mix equal quantities of powdered sage leaves (*Salvia officinalis*) and sugar. Take every morning before breakfast for several weeks.

Sucker Fish Gall

For fits, take the gall of a sucker fish (family Catostomidae) 2 or 3 times a day.

Comments

None of these remedies has any proven merit in the treatment of convulsive illness of any kind.

⤳Foot Problems⤶ (Corns, Calluses, Ingrown Toenails)

Bacon

For an ingrown toenail, apply a piece of raw bacon and allow to remain overnight.

Castor Oil

To remove corns from the feet, just dab a little castor oil on them daily. After about ten days, they will simply peel off.

Water, Vinegar

Corns and calluses may be softened by soaking the feet in hot soapy water to which a cup of cider vinegar has been added.

Comments

Corns and calluses are locally hardened or thickened areas of the skin. Both the castor oil treatment and the hot water-vinegar treatment would serve to soften them and aid in their removal. The fat in raw bacon will also soften the skin around an ingrown toenail, thereby reducing the pain and allowing the nail to grow out normally.

⇨Frostbite⇦

Beech Leaves

To help frostbite, boiled beech tree leaves (*Fagus grandiflora*) are folded into a white cotton cloth and placed as a poultice on the affected area for 1 hour.

Oak Leaves

Collect oak leaves that have remained on the tree during the winter and boil them in water to make a strong tea. Soak the feet in this for 1 hour several nights in a row.

> *The feet did not pain after using the tea.*
> Mildred Dively

Comments

Freezing of the superficial tissues produces the condition known as frostbite. It results in more or less structural damage accompanied by some loss of function of the small surface blood vessels. The condition is best treated by rapid thawing at temperatures just slightly above body heat. This minimizes destruction of the tissues.

The treatments reported here would be initially somewhat useful in thawing the afflicted parts, providing they are applied warm and not hot. In addition, the contained tannins would provide a slight antiseptic action. The warm baths or poultices would also tend to stimulate circulation and thereby promote healing.

⇒Gout⇐

Wild Cherries

Eat ½ cupful of wild black cherries (*Prunus serotina*) or choke-cherries (*Prunus virginiana*) daily to cure gout.

> *This was a very successful treatment.* Mary Willets

Comments

Acidic fruits, especially black currants, juniper berries, plums, and cherries, have the reputation of helping to break down and promote the excretion of uric acid which is the cause of gout. It would seem that any of the aforementioned would be easier to obtain and better tasting than the extremely tart wild cherries recommended by our informant. All of the sources, including this one, indicate that regular consumption of the fruits is required to obtain satisfactory results.

⇒Headache⇐

Boneset

Boneset (*Eupatorium perfoliatum*) is recommended for migraine. Drink when you feel the symptoms coming on.

Camphor

Rub camphor spirits on the forehead to cure a headache.

Ground Ivy

Ground ivy tea (*Glechoma hederacea*) will cure a headache.

Horseradish

Placed bruised horseradish leaves (*Armoracia rusticana*) on the forehead for headache.

Indian Turnip

Indian turnip (*Arisaema triphyllum*) is a useful remedy for headache.

Northern Prickly Ash

Use finely powdered root bark from the northern prickly ash (*Zanthoxylum americanum*) as a snuff to cure a headache.

Pennyroyal

Drink pennyroyal tea (*Hedeoma pulegioides*) with a little sugar in it to cure sick (migraine) headache.

Sage, Rosemary

Tea made from sage leaves (*Salvia officinalis*) with a pinch of rosemary (*Rosmarinus officinalis*) gives quick headache relief.

Spider Web

A headache can be cured by swallowing a spider web.

Trumpet Weed

The stalks of trumpet weed or joe-pye-weed (*Eupatorium* spp.) are used as an herb tea to cure headache.

Vinegar

Soak brown paper or a cloth in vinegar and apply to the fore-head to cure a headache.

Vinegar

Mix equal parts of water and vinegar, place in a saucepan, and bring to a boil. Inhale the vapor for 75 breaths. This will stop migraine headache.

Water

Apply hot water on a cloth to the forehead for headache.

Water

Apply cold water on a cloth to the back of the neck to relieve a dull headache.

Willow Twigs

To relieve a headache, chew willow twigs (*Salix* spp.) until your ears ring.

Yellow Ladyslipper

To obtain relief from a headache, the roots of the yellow lady-slipper (*Cypripedium calceolus*) are dug fresh, cleansed well, and allowed to lie in the sun and fresh air for an hour. Make a medium-strength tea with boiling water. Use no more than twice a day.

Comments

Willow twigs contain salicin (salicyl alcohol glucoside), a compound related chemically to aspirin and one that produces similar analgesic effects. Chewing the twigs might cure a headache, but you will have to chew a lot of them before your ears begin to ring. Doses of salicylates in excess of 10 grams daily (equivalent to about 30 regular-sized aspirin tablets) do cause toxic effects, including tinnitus or ringing in the ears. This is equal to the amount of salicin in a pound or more of most willow barks. It is quite unlikely that anyone would chew this quantity of plant material.

Application of water, hot or cold, or of a rubefacient, such as camphor, to the forehead or neck may influence the degree of dilation or constriction of the blood vessels in those regions and thus modify certain types of headache. The inhalation of vinegar fumes (acetic acid) will certainly cause a person to think about something other than a headache. The same applies to snuffing powdered prickly ash bark. Based on present knowledge, the claims made for the other remedies do not appear to have basis in fact.

Heat Exhaustion

Mayapple Fruits

Eat mayapple fruits (*Podophyllum peltatum*) to help overcome heat exhaustion.

Comments

Although the roots of mayapple act as a powerful purgative, the fruits are perfectly edible and delicious as well. Eating them would tend to restore some of the salts (electrolytes) to the body which are lost in the profuse sweating accompanying heat exhaustion. Also the sugars in them would serve as a source of energy. Many other edible fruits would probably serve the same function just as effectively.

⤳Hemorrhoids⤳ (Piles)

Ben-Gay

Apply Ben-Gay (Methyl salicylate and menthol ointment).

One night, in the dark, I accidentally used Ben-Gay instead of Preparation H. At the time, it was extremely uncomfortable, but the effect continues to amaze me. That was at least twenty years ago, but believe it or not, I have not been troubled with hemorrhoids ever since. Anonymous

(Note: This painful remedy is not recommended. See compiler's comments.)

Horse Chestnuts

Horse chestnut ointment: Remove the shells from 6 horse chestnuts (*Aesculus hippocastanum*) and chop the nutmeats very fine. Cover the nuts with lard and warm gently for 1 hour. Cool and apply to the affected parts twice daily.

This is a very valuable remedy for piles. Doris Tilghman

Jimson Weed

Hemorrhoids are effectively treated by applying a salve made from bruised jimson weed leaves (*Datura stramonium*) mixed with lard.

Turpentine

For hemorrhoids, mix turpentine oil with lard or unsalted butter and apply as needed.

(Note: This painful remedy is not recommended. See compiler's comments.)

Comments

Horse chestnut extract is widely used in Europe in ointments and soaps of various kinds intended to minimize the effects of varicose veins. It is also a very common ingredient there in preparations (ointments, suppositories) intended for the treatment of hemorrhoids. Consequently, the horse chestnut ointment may indeed be, as the correspondent indicates, a "valuable remedy for piles."

Jimson weed ointment might possibly exert some desirable antispasmodic effect on the smooth muscles of the lower bowel, and belladonna extract, with its similar active constituents (primarily atropine), is incorporated into certain commercial hemorrhoid preparations. However, such drugs are quite toxic and absorption from the diseased skin and irritated rectal mucosa of the user might be excessive. Use of jimson weed in the local treatment of hemorrhoids is no longer considered rational.

The use of turpentine spirits is almost as heroic and would certainly be nearly as painful as the accidental application of Ben-Gay (methyl salicylate and menthol ointment) which the anonymous contributor found to be so effective. Needless to say, both of these latter treatments would be excessively painful and irritating. They cannot, therefore, be recommended.

⇒Hiccups⇐

Dillseed

Chew dillseed (*Anethum graveolens*) or sip tea made from it to relieve the hiccups.

Fright

Scare the sufferer to stop the hiccups.

Hold Breath

To cure the hiccups, hold the breath as long as possible.

Peanut Butter

Eat a teaspoonful of peanut butter to cure the hiccups.

Sugar

Eat sugar to relieve the hiccups.

Sulfur

To cure the hiccups, swallow a small lump of sulfur.

Water

Sip water repeatedly without taking a breath to treat hiccups.

Water

Stop the hiccups by taking 9 sips of water, 3 at a time.

Comments

Hiccups are spasmodic inhalations of air accompanied by closure of the glottis or space between the vocal cords. Probably all of the above treatments are somewhat useful in stopping the spasms which are responsible for them.

↭Hives and Allergic Skin Reactions↭

Ground Ivy

To relieve the hives, drink tea made from ground ivy (*Glechoma hederacea*).

Nightshade

Wash and boil the leaves of nightshade (*Solanum nigrum*) in a small amount of water until tender. Add a few teaspoonfuls of cornmeal to thicken. Spoon it onto a clean cloth and fold it in. Apply to the affected area while warm and leave in place for 1 hour. The poultice is very effective for hives and allergic rashes.

Red Alder

Tea made from red alder bark (*Alnus* spp.) is drunk to cure hives.

Red Alder

The leaves and bark of the red alder (*Alnus* spp.) brewed into a strong tea will help the hives. It is applied locally to the affected area and 2 tablespoonfuls are also taken internally. Repeat every hour until relieved.

Comments

None of these remedies possesses any antihistaminic activity which would cause it to be especially useful in treating the hives and similar allergic skin reactions. Thus, the suggested medications are purely palliative in their effects. Red alder is an astringent which would help relieve itching when applied locally. Nightshade is widely recommended by practitioners of folk medicine for a variety of skin conditions.

⇾Hunger⇽

Elm Leaves

Eat elm leaves (*Ulmus americana*) to relieve hunger pangs.

> *Of all the tree leaves, these are the best for this purpose.* N. Davidson

Comments

Elm leaves do not contain any large quantities of nutrients that are readily assimilable by human beings. Thus, their purported ability to relieve hunger, if factual, must be attributed to other constituents which have not yet been identified.

❧Insect Bites and Stings❧

Ammonia Water

Swabbing on household ammonia water with a piece of cotton will help a bee sting.

Baking Soda

Apply baking soda, moistened to a paste, to relieve insect bites or stings.

Borax

Borax dissolved in a little water will alleviate the pain of bee and wasp stings.

Chewing Tobacco

Application of a moist wad of chewing tobacco directly to the affected area will relieve the pain of bee stings.

Dock Leaves

Rub dock leaves (*Rumex* spp.) on a bee sting to relieve the pain.

Houseleek

A green salve made by rendering the leaves of houseleek (*Sempervivium tectorum*) in lard is good for insect stings and bites.

Meat Tenderizer

A relatively recent cure for insect stings is the application of moist meat tenderizer (papain) to the affected area.

Mud

Apply mud to a bee sting or insect bite to relieve the discomfort.

Nightshade

The nightshade poultice described in the section Poison Ivy and Poison Sumac is also said to be effective for bee stings.

Onion

The pain from bee or wasp stings is relieved by the application of either scraped onion or simply a slice of onion. This treatment is also effective for dog bite.

Plantain

For quick relief from the pain of a bee sting, rub it with a plantain leaf (*Plantago* spp.).

Plantain

Drink the fresh juice squeezed from green plantain leaves (*Plantago* spp.), and apply the leaves themselves to the affected area to cure the bite of a venomous spider.

Raw Meat

The pain from the sting of a bee or wasp may be relieved almost instantly by applying a piece of lean raw meat to the affected area.

Rhubarb Juice

Juice from a broken rhubarb stock (*Rheum rhaponticum*) will help relieve the pain of an insect bite.

Salt, Baking Soda

Mix salt and baking soda in equal parts, add a little water and apply to bee and wasp stings.

Sulfur, Lard

Mix sulfur and lard to make an ointment that is an effective chigger repellant and that also relieves the itching of the bites.

Weeds (Four Kinds)

When stung by a bee, take four different kinds of weeds (any kind of weeds) and rub them together until you get a juice. Rub this juice on the bee sting and it will take out the pain.

Weeds (Three Kinds)

As above, but use only three different kinds of weeds.

Comments

Household therapy for insect bites and stings most often seems to involve the application of an alkaline material, of something moist, or of some kind of plant juice or extract. In the first category are found baking soda (or salt and soda), borax, and ammonia water. Moist materials include, as always, onion slices or scrapings, plus chewing tobacco, mud, and raw meat. Plant juices embrace those of dock, houseleek, nightshade, the ever-useful plantain, rhubarb, and, as a matter of fact, a combination of any three or four different weeds chosen at random.

Just how well these various agents work is problematic. Probably all provide some relief from a painful or irritating condition that is often quite transient anyway. By the time one has located four different weeds, for example, the bite or sting has probably ceased to be acutely painful.

Meat tenderizers are composed primarily of papain, an enzyme obtained from papaya fruits, that has the ability to hydrolyze not only protein but some carbohydrates and fats as well. The rationale in applying it to an insect sting is that the pain-producing venom is proteinaceous in nature. On contact with the enzyme, it will be rapidly destroyed, and the pain will be eliminated.

In my experience, sulfur is a much more effective chigger repellant than it is a treatment for their bites. Nevertheless, the sulfur-lard combination may provide some relief from their persistent itching.

⇒Insect Repellants⇐

Black Walnut Leaves

To prepare a useful insect repellant, take 2 or 3 handfuls of fresh black walnut leaves (*Juglans nigra*) and let soak overnight in 2 or 3 quarts of water. Boil for 15 minutes and allow to cool. Apply with a sponge. This is useful for horses or people. A person can also rub the fresh walnut leaves directly on the skin.

Borax, Red Pepper

A mixture of borax and red pepper sprinkled on shelves will drive ants away.

Pennyroyal

Hang up bunches of pennyroyal plants (*Hedeoma pulegioides*) to drive away mosquitoes.

Sassafras

Sprinkle sassafras root (*Sassafras albidum*) around doors and windows to keep out ants.

Shoo-Fly

The shoo-fly plant (*Nicandra physalodes*) will keep flies away.

Sweet Wormwood

Sweet wormwood (*Artemesia annua*) develops a very pronounced and pleasant fragrance when the plant dries. It will keep away moths and other insects.

Comments

It is well-known that many plant materials, particularly those containing odoriferous volatile oils, have the ability to repel insects. Those listed here are probably all more or less effective. Black walnut leaves are noted as being especially useful. It is sometimes recommended that a branch of them be hung in the bedroom to keep out gnats and mosquitoes.

One plant that is occasionally used, but which fortunately was not recommended by any of my sources, is rue or garden rue (*Ruta graveolens*). When applied to the skin—the leaves are ordinarily rubbed on—certain constituents in its volatile oil react with sunlight to produce photosensitization. This results in a very painful rash accompanied by blisters. Obviously, the use of rue in this manner is definitely not recommended.

⇗Jaundice and Hepatitis⇖

Deer Horns

Make and drink tea from powdered deer horns for jaundice.

Egg Yolk

The yolk of an egg, either raw or slightly cooked, is an excellent food for jaundice.

Herbal Mixture

To cure jaundice, take sarsaparilla roots (*Smilax* spp.), red sumac (*Rhus glabra*), bitter root (*Apocynum androsaemifolium*), wild cherry bark (*Prunus serotina*), and wild poplar roots (*Liriodendron tulipifera*) and boil together in water. Strain, and mix the extract with hard cider and a little more water. Take ½ teacupful 3 times a day.

Jack Oak Ashes, Potassium Bicarbonate, Pokeberry Juice

To cure jaundice, use a poultice made from jack oak ashes (*Quercus ellipsoidalis*), saleratus (potassium or sodium bicarbonate), and pokeberry juice (*Phytolacca americana*).

Liverwort

Make tea from the leaves of liverwort (*Hepatica* spp.) to cure liver problems—jaundice and hepatitis.

Onions, Molasses, Cornmeal

For jaundice, apply a poultice of boiled onions, molasses, and cornmeal.

Pumpkin Seeds

Boiled pumpkin seeds are eaten to cure jaundice.

Sow Bugs

For yellow jaundice, collect five or six large sow bugs (genus *Oniscus*) from under rotten logs and boil them in a small amount of water. Drink the resulting broth.

Wild Cherry Bark

Drink a tea made from wild cherry bark (*Prunus serotina*) to cure yellow jaundice.

Wild Cherry Bark, Peach Tree Bark

Drink tea made from wild cherry bark (*Prunus serotina*) and peach tree bark (*Prunus persica*) to cure jaundice.

Comments

Since jaundice and the hepatitis that often causes it are ordinarily very serious conditions, the innocuous remedies reported here are unlikely to be of any use in treating them. The liverwort tea is obviously based on the long-discredited doctrine of signatures which held that plants or plant parts resembling various organs of the body were useful in treating diseases of those organs. Thus, liverwort was thought to be effective for diseases of the liver, namely, jaundice and hepatitis.

All of the other remedies are equally fanciful, at least in terms of any proven therapeutic utility. Note once again, however, the appearance of an onion poultice.

⋙Kidney Problems⋘

Alder

For dropsy (edema), boil the small white roots of alder (*Alnus* spp.) in water and drink the liquid.

Asparagus

A useful diuretic is made by bruising or shredding the roots of asparagus (*Asparagus officinalis*) and soaking them in cold water. Drink this beverage frequently throughout the day.

Bearberry

A tea from bearberry leaves (*Arctostaphylos uva-ursi*) is a useful diuretic.

Corn Silks

Tea made from corn silks (*Zea mays*) will flush out your kidneys.

Cream of Tartar

Take ¼ teaspoonful of cream of tartar dissolved in a glass of water as a diuretic and for albumin in the urine.

Elder Bark

Simmer the bark of the elder (*Sambucus canadensis*) in wine for an hour. Strain and bottle. Drink ½ cupful daily to expel fluid and relieve dropsy.

Goldenrod

Tea made from the flowers, leaves, and stalk of common goldenrod (*Solidago* spp.) is used to treat bladder inflammation.

Honeylocust

Tea made from the roots of the honeylocust (*Gleditsia triacanthos*) is effective for kidney trouble.

Indian Turnip

To increase the flow of urine, drink Indian turnip root (*Arisaema triphyllum*) boiled in sweet milk.

Onion Juice, Horsemint

To dissolve kidney stones, drink a teacupful of red onion juice and a pint of horsemint tea (*Monarda punctata*) twice a day, morning and evening. Drink the 2 beverages separately; do not mix them together. The effects will be noted within 3 days.

Pumpkin Seeds

Eat the kernels from pumpkin seeds for kidney trouble.

Queen-of-the-Meadow

Boil the flowers of queen-of-the-meadow (*Eupatorium purpureum*) in water and add sugar to make a drink for kidney ailments.

Stone Root

The root of horsebalm or stoneroot (*Collinsonia canadensis*) is given for kidney stones.

Sycamore Buds, Whiskey

Allow 1 ounce of sycamore buds (*Platanus occidentalis*) to digest in a pint of whiskey for 1 week with frequent shaking. Take 1 to 2 teaspoonfuls as a diuretic.

Watermelon (Seeds)

Eat watermelon or drink tea made from the seeds to cure kidney trouble.

White Sassafras

Tea made from the white sassafras (*Sassafras albidum*) is a remedy for kidney trouble.

White Snakeroot

Drink tea made from white snakeroot (*Eupatorium rugosum*) for kidney problems. (Note: Extremely poisonous. Do not use!)

Comments

Generally, when kidney problems are referred to, the informant is discussing the need for a diuretic, that is, something to increase the flow of urine. Although not strictly a problem of the kidneys, dropsy is a condition involving accumulation of fluid in the tissues and is often treated, at least in part, with a diuretic. Therefore, it, too, is included in this category. Other kidney problems include diseases resulting in albumin in the urine (Bright's disease), kidney stones, and various kidney and urinary tract infections. Even prostatitis may be included in the broad category, and pumpkin seeds, which have been widely promoted recently for that condition, were recommended by one source as a cure for "kidney trouble."

Among the listed remedies that have long been recognized for their diuretic properties are bearberry, corn silk, elder bark, queen-of-the-meadow, white sassafras, and watermelon seeds. Some of the other herbs may also promote the formation and excretion of urine. Cream of tartar (potassium bitartrate) is also a known diuretic, but it certainly will not cure cases involving albumin in the urine.

Neither will stone root nor red onion juice and horsemint tea relieve kidney stones. Large volumes of liquid are, of course, helpful, but these herbal remedies will not otherwise facilitate the passage of stones through the ureters.

The white snakeroot tea that one correspondent suggested for kidney trouble should never be used internally, for the plant is extremely poisonous. In the early days in Indiana, when cattle were often allowed to roam the woods, milk cows sometimes ate it. People drinking the milk from these cows acquired the so-called trembles or milk sickness, with sometimes fatal results. Nancy Hanks Lincoln, Abraham's mother, died of the milk sickness in Spencer County in 1818.

⇒Lice and "The Itch"⇐

Kerosene

Apply kerosene to affected area to kill "cooties" (body lice).

Pokeroot

A soothing salve to relieve the itch is made from pokeroots (*Phytolacca americana*). These are dug, washed, allowed to dry, and then ground or chopped very fine. Mix with lard or vaseline to make a salve. This is applied to the affected area several times a day.

Pokeroot

Relieve the itch by bathing the affected area in water in which pokeroots (*Phytolacca americana*) have been boiled.

Sulfur, Lard

Mix sulfur and lard and rub thoroughly into the hair to kill head lice.

Sulfur, Lard

Make an ointment of sulfur and lard to cure the itch.

Comments

Although lice and "the itch" are not the the same, the result—an intense itching sensation—caused by both, as well as the listed treatments for both, are similar. Indeed, in pioneer days the conditions were often referred to in the same breath.

A louse is a small, wingless, flattened, sucking insect (*Pediculus humanis*) that feeds on the body (body louse) or often on the scalp (head louse) of human beings. The itch, on the other hand, is a contagious skin eruption caused by a mite (*Sarcoptes scabiei*) that burrows in the skin.

Before the mid-twentieth century, development of effective, synthetic chemical pediculicides (lice killers) and miticides (mite killers), these conditions were very difficult to treat. The information supplied notes the use of kerosene or sulfur salve to kill lice. The latter remedy, as well as pokeroot salve or water extract, was also applied to the itch.

In the absence of careful personal hygiene, these treatments were probably ineffective or, at the best, temporary. Because of their toxicity, pokeroot preparations cannot be recommended, even for external use.

⋙Malaria⋘

American Centaury

The American centaury plant (*Sabatia angularis*) is widely used as an ingredient in bitter teas and extracts used to treat the ague (malaria). For this reason, in Indiana, it is sometimes called ague weed. This should not be confused with boneset (*Eupatorium perfoliatium*) which is also commonly called ague weed.

Dogwood Bark

Dogwood bark (*Cornus florida*) is taken to cure malaria.

Ironweed

To cure malaria, boil the roots of ironweed (*Veronia* spp.) in water and drink the resulting extract.

Queen-of-the-Meadow; Boneset

Indiana pioneers used queen-of-the-meadow (*Eupatorium purpureum*) to treat malaria, but they preferred for this purpose the closely related plant, boneset (*Eupatorium perfoliatum*).

Comments

Other than having the ability to cause sweating and thereby moderate somewhat the fever associated with malaria, all of the remedies noted for the treatment of this disease are ineffective. They do possess an additional feature in common, namely, their bitterness. This property probably reminded early-day herbalists of the bitter taste of cinchona bark (quinine) which was effective in treating malaria, and they wrongly assumed these plant materials would be equally useful.

❧Measles❧

Corn Silk

Drink hot corn silk tea (*Zea mays*) to help measles rash to develop.

Dandelion Wine

Drink dandelion wine (*Taraxacum officinale*) to promote the development of measles rash and to lessen the severity of the disease.

> *The remedy given me was large quantities of dandelion wine. I did break out, and I suspect the initial phase of the disease was less difficult because I was drunk for some time.* Mary Stevens

Ginger

Drink hot ginger tea to help measles rash to develop.

Mullein

Drink hot mullein leaf tea (*Verbascum thapsus*) to help measles rash to develop.

Sage

Drink hot sage tea (*Salvia officinalis*) to help measles rash to develop.

Sassafras

Hot sassafras tea (*Sassafras albidum*) will "bring out" the measles.

Sheep Dung

Drink hot tea made from sheep dung to help the measles "break out."

Sheep Dung

Place dried sheep dung in a cloth bag, boil in water, and drink the liquid to make measles "break out."

Spicebush

Drink hot spicebush tea (*Benzoin aestivale*) to help measles rash to develop.

Wild Cherry

To relieve some of the discomfort associated with measles, drink tea made from the bark of the wild cherry tree (*Prunus serotina*).

Comments

Once the typical rash develops, that is, once the measles "break out," it is a well-known fact that the patient feels much better. Various herbal teas and related preparations are recommended by informants to promote this process by causing abundant perspiration. Their efficacy in hastening onset of the rash is questionable, although, with the exception of sheep dung and sassafras, they are not harmful. The former is unsanitary; the latter is toxic. See comments following the section Blood Thinners, Purifiers, and Tonics.

Sage tea, although recommended by one source, would not promote perspiration, but instead, would hinder it. Its value therefore seems especially doubtful.

✒Menstrual Problems✒

Chamomile

Drink chamomile tea (*Anthemis nobilis*) for menstrual cramps.

Ginger

Drink sweetened ginger tea to relieve menstrual cramps.

Ginger

Drinking hot ginger tea will bring on delayed menstruation.

Wintergreen, Sugar

For menstrual cramps, mix wintergreen oil with sugar and take with water.

Comments

All of the agents listed have the reputation of acting as emmenagogues or menstrual stimulants. In addition, chamomile is noted for its antispasmodic properties which are claimed to be especially effective against menstrual cramps.

❧Nausea and Vomiting❧

Charcoal

To check vomiting, place several big chunks of charcoal in a pan of water and let it stand awhile. Drain off the water and give 1½ teaspoonfuls every 5 to 10 minutes for nausea and vomiting.

Peach Tree Bark

A tea made from peach tree bark (*Prunus persica*) will overcome nausea.

Peppermint

Eat peppermint candy to cure nausea.

Popcorn

To relieve nausea, pop some popcorn without using grease and place in a bowl. Pour in enough boiling water to cover the corn. Cover and let stand for 15 minutes. Take 1 teaspoonful every 10 minutes.

Salt, Red Pepper, Vinegar

The best remedy to stop vomiting is to take a heaping teaspoonful each of salt and red pepper, and add a teacupful of vinegar. Take 1 tablespoonful every 15 to 30 minutes as needed.

Sheep Sorrel, Wild Mint

For nausea, drink the water extract of sheep sorrel and wild mint described in the section Stomachache and Colic.

Vinegar

Morning sickness can be prevented by drinking 1 teaspoonful of apple cider vinegar dissolved in a glass of water.

Wild Mint

Eat boiled wild mint leaves (*Blephilia, Monarda,* and *Pycnanthemum* spp.) to cure nausea.

Comments

Normally, it is assumed that vomiting or the tendency to vomit is best checked by agents that either facilitate digestion and cause excess gas to be expelled or by those that soothe and allay the existing irritation of the stomach. This is reflected in the submitted remedies that involve mints, which do serve as carminatives (agents that expel gas) and the charcoal water with its adsorbent properties as well as the popcorn water with its content of starch and sugars; the water involved is also helpful in maintaining adequate hydration.

But this logic is not followed in the case of the vinegar treatment for morning sickness and, especially, the salt, red pepper, and vinegar recipe which is advanced as a sovereign remedy for vomiting. Assuming that these do actually work, it would appear that at least certain materials capable of irritating the stomach lining also are effective against nausea and vomiting. If they are not effective, they are at least well-known. I was so skeptical about including them in this section that I checked other compilations of folkloric remedies and found salt and vinegar as well as red pepper all listed as agents recommended for the relief of nausea.

Although ginger was not included in the recipes submitted by Hoosier informants, recent clinical studies have shown that it is effective in preventing motion sickness. Since it, too, is quite pungent, perhaps the pungency of both red pepper and vinegar causes these products to produce a similar effect. The entire matter needs further study before a satisfactory explanation can be given.

❧Nervousness and Insomnia❧

Catnip

Catnip tea (*Nepeta cataria*) is given to fussy babies to quiet them. It is also a useful sedative for adults.

Catnip

Boil catnip (*Nepeta cataria*) leaves in water and add sugar to make a syrup. Give to babies to make them sleep.

Celery

Eat celery to overcome nervousness.

Garlic

Steep 2 cloves of garlic in hot water, allow to cool, and drink.

You will sleep good. Margie M. Fogleman

Honey

Eat honey to promote sound sleep.

Hops

Drink hot tea made from hops (*Humulus* spp.) to make one sleep. Using a pillow filled with hops is also helpful.

Ladyslipper, Ginseng, Nutmeg

Steep some pulverized ladyslipper (*Cypripedium* spp.) and about half as much ginseng (*Panax quinquefolius*) together with a little nutmeg in hot water. Sip as needed to calm the nerves.

Onions

Eat a quantity of onions as an effective tranquilizer.

Onions, Salt

A raw onion, eaten with a little salt, will often produce sleep in a few minutes.

Red Sumac

Tea prepared from the dried berries of red sumac (*Rhus glabra*) calms the nerves. Be sure to strain out the fine hairs.

Sage

Sage (*Salvia officinalis*) tea is a useful remedy for sleeplessness.

Sweet Anise

Tea of sweet anise (*Osmorhiza longistylis*) is a useful calmative.

Tulip Tree

Tea made from the blossoms of the tulip tree (*Liriodendron tulipifera*) is a useful calmative in cases of hysteria.

Valerian

Put 4 ounces of pulverized valerian root (*Valeriana officinalis*) in a pint of alcohol in a closed bottle. Let it stand in the hot sun for about 10 days, shaking frequently. Strain or filter and take 1 to 3 teaspoonfuls as needed. The remedy is a valuable one for all nervous symptoms.

Water

To promote sleep, wet a cloth in cold water and place it on the back of the neck. Cover with a smooth towel and lie down.

Wild Lettuce

Wild lettuce leaves (*Lactuca scariola*) are a readily available substitute for opium. They have a mild sedative effect.

Comments

Those who think that the use of tranquilizers and sedatives is associated exclusively with our modern, high-tech society need only to look at the number of treatments for nervousness and insomnia utilized as traditional home remedies to realize that the need for such medicines is not restricted to the present day. Some of the recipes listed are probably quite useful, although scientific proof of their effectiveness is scanty at best.

Catnip was mentioned more frequently by informants than any other product in this category, being especially recommended by them for infants. A recent subjective test of sedative teas published in a popular magazine found catnip to be the most efficacious.

Valerian has a thousand-year-old history as a minor tranquilizer and calmative. Scores of pharmaceutical products containing valerian are available in Europe at the present time. Scientific research has shown that valerian does have some activity, but the active principles are quite unstable. Whether they would exist in any quantity in the alcoholic preparation described is problematic. A tea made from the fresh roots would probably be more effective.

Hops is another herbal product demonstrated to possess some sedative activity. At least one of the active principles in it is volatile, so the utility of a hop pillow in promoting sleep cannot be completely discounted.

The dried milky juice (latex) of wild lettuce, often referred to as lettuce opium, has been used since the time of the ancient Egyptians for its sleep-producing properties. Research has shown that the fresh latex does contain certain bitter principles capable of producing depressant or sedative effects. Since these were absent in the dried material, only fresh wild lettuce leaves should be employed.

Garlic and the omnipresent onion are both present in the listing of useful sleep promoters. A number of sources testify to their effectiveness, and my own father was a strong believer in the soporific properties of raw onions.

Any effectiveness of the remaining remedies is much less certain. Ladyslipper has an unverified reputation as a narcotic, but ginseng, with which it is combined in the listed recipe, is basically a stimulant. Preparing any hot tea, then sitting down and slowly consuming it, probably has beneficial calmative effects. The same may be said for the application of a cold compress to the back of the neck followed by the assumption of a horizontal position. The latter act alone is often conducive to sleep in many individuals.

⇨Nettle Burn⇦

Dock Leaves

Rub dock leaves (*Rumex* spp.) on nettle burn to relieve the itching.

Comments

I, personally, count it a tragedy that a society capable of splitting the atom and of enabling men to walk and ride on the surface of the moon is unable to state with certainty the cause of the pain and irritation resulting from contact with the stinging nettle. But such is the case, in spite of the fact that nettles have been around for a long time.

Indeed, so have the cures for so-called nettle burn. One of the oldest is rubbing with dock leaves, as noted in the ancient rhyme:

"Nettle in, dock out.
Dock rub nettle out!"

No one knows how this works either, if indeed it does. Rubbing alone seems to have some beneficial effect in relieving nettle burn. Also the time involved in searching out a dock leaf may be sufficient to allow the irritation to subside somewhat.

⟩Neuritis and Neuralgia⟨

Bull Thistle

The worst case of neuralgia that ever existed can be permanently cured by drinking a tea and applying a poultice made from the leaves of the bull thistle (*Cirsium vulgare*).

Figs, Raisins, etc.

Recipe for neuritis cure:

Figs	1.5 pound
Seedless raisins	1 box
Olive oil	1.5 fluid ounce
Glycerin	0.5 fluid ounce
Powdered senna (*Cassia* spp.)	1.5 ounce
Slippery elm (*Ulmus fulva*)	0.5 ounce
Powdered charcoal	1 ounce

Grind the figs and raisins together and add the other ingredients. Mix well and form into balls the size of small walnuts. Keep refrigerated. Take (chew) 1 ball morning and evening for a week; then take 1 a day for 6 months.

Vinegar

Facial neuralgia is relieved by taking 1 teaspoonful of cider vinegar in a glass of water.

Comments

There is little reason to believe that any of these remedies would have a beneficial effect on the cause or symptoms of either neuritis or neuralgia. The figs, raisins, etc., recipe is a rather potent laxative, and if used as directed, it would divert one's attention from any discomfort caused by neuritis. A moist poultice of any kind might bring some relief from neuralgia.

❧Nosebleed❧

Coin

A nosebleed can be stopped by holding a penny or a dime to the roof of your mouth with your tongue.

Coin (Penny)

To stop a nosebleed place a penny between the upper teeth and lip. Hold there for a few minutes.

Cold Metal; Ice

To stop a nosebleed, hold a cold knife, a key, a pair of scissors, or a piece of ice on the back of the person's neck.

Cold Water

Dip the hands in cold water to cure a nosebleed.

Horseradish

Pulverize horseradish root (*Armoracia rusticana*) and use as a snuff for nosebleed.

Metal

Place a door key or a pair of scissors on the person's chest to cure a nosebleed.

Paper

Hold a piece of paper under the upper lip to cure a nosebleed.

Paper, Vinegar

To cure a nosebleed hold a piece of brown paper soaked in vinegar under the upper lip.

Pressure

Simply press on the upper lip to cure a nosebleed.

Red Pepper, Hot Water

Stop a nosebleed by bathing the feet in very hot water and, at the same time, drinking a pint of cayenne (red) pepper tea.

Silver

Hold a piece of silver under the upper lip to stop a nosebleed.

Witch Hazel Leaves

To stop a nosebleed, crumble up dry witch hazel leaves (*Hamamelis virginiana*) and stuff them up your nose.

Comments

Those remedies involving metal or paper held in the mouth or applied to some part of the anatomy (neck, chest) seem to fall more in the realm of magic or charms than in that of medicine. Nevertheless, because they are somewhat borderline cases and because they were suggested by so many correspondents, they are included here.

Using snuff made from powdered horseradish root would seem to be an extremely irritating measure with more detrimental than beneficial effects. It is certainly not recommended. Witch hazel leaves, on the other hand, possess valuable astringent properties due to their contained tannins and would appear to be a useful remedy. The hot footbath-red pepper tea treatment would draw some blood away from the head, thus lessening the tendency to nosebleed, but the amount involved would not be very significant. Many persons would find drinking a pint of red pepper tea more unpleasant than having a slight nosebleed.

⤳Perspiration Odor⤶

Ammonia Water

Wash with a solution of 2 tablespoonfuls of household ammonia in water to prevent perspiration odor.

Comments

Household ammonia is an effective detergent. It should be sufficiently diluted so as not to irritate the skin.

⤳Pleurisy⤶

Butterflyweed

The root of butterflyweed or pleurisy root (*Asclepias tuberosa*) is, as the latter common name implies, used to treat pleurisy.

Comments

Butterflyweed has the reputation of relaxing the capillary blood vessels, thereby relieving the strain on heart and lungs. This, in turn, is supposed to relieve pain and make breathing easier in cases of pleurisy. Scientific evidence for these reputed effects is lacking.

⇒Pneumonia⇐

Onions, Rye Meal, Vinegar

To cure pneumonia, fry 6 to 10 chopped onions in a large frying pan together with an equal quantity of rye meal and enough vinegar to make a thick paste. Stir continually while simmering for 5 to 10 minutes. Put in a cotton bag and apply very hot to the patient's chest. Replace with a similar hot poultice when it begins to cool. Repeat 3 or 5 times until perspiration starts from chest.

This never fails. It has been used successfully after physicians have given up. Anonymous

Comments

Once again, we have a recommendation for the ever-popular onion poultice for chest complaint—this time pneumonia. See comments in the section Colds and Flu.

❧Poison Ivy and Poison Sumac Dermatitis❧

Copperas, Sugar of Lead

Apply a solution of copperas (ferrous sulfate) or of sugar of lead (lead acetate) to cure poison ivy rash.

Deadly Nightshade

Juice from the leaves or ripe berries of deadly nightshade (*Atropa belladonna*) is rubbed on the skin to reduce poison ivy rash.

Elder Root

An extract made by boiling elder root (*Sambucus canadensis*) in water is rubbed lightly on the affected area to cure poison ivy rash.

Hemlock

Bathe poison ivy rash in water in which hemlock twigs or leaves (*Tsuga canadensis*) have been steeped.

Houseleek

To cure poison ivy or poison sumac rash, pick some leaves of the houseleek (*Sempervivum tectorum*) and mash them between the fingers so as to rupture the back membranes of them. Rub the juice on the affected area. Although it will be coated with a green film, the rash will get better, almost immediately.

> *Taught me by my grandmother, Mrs. Ruth A. Hillenburg.* Joyce M. Kelley

Jewelweed

Jewelweed or wild touch-me-not (*Impatiens* spp.) is best used to treat poison ivy in the following way. The plant is cut a few inches above ground level and the stem is then slit lengthwise with a penknife. A gluey juice (not unlike that of okra) is emitted, and this is rubbed directly on the affected area. Do not try to transfer the juice onto the finger to apply, just rub the inside of the stem itself on the area and let it dry. Do not rinse for several hours. This works best before flowering. After that occurs, the juice is not as plentiful.

> *Jewelweed juice is useful in both treating and preventing poison ivy. Unprotected areas of skin may be treated with it in anticipation of ivy contact. It is also useful for minor cuts and for insect bites. My husband and I have both received relief by using it on many occasions.*
> Barbara Fluegeman

Jewelweed

To cure poison ivy rash or to help develop an immunity against it, boil jewelweed (*Impatiens* spp.) in water and drink the liquid. Any part of the plant—root, stem, leaves, or flowers—can be used. Drink a couple of times during the summer just to develop your resistance. Alternatively, you can eat jewelweed greens made by cooking a couple of cups of the leaves in a little water.

> *It has worked for me. I used to get ivy rash very badly, with big watery blisters, but after a couple of years of this treatment, I would only get a rash that wasn't weepy. Now I do not get the rash, although I frequently mow in it since moving to the country.* Doris Parks

Jewelweed

Strip the leaves from jewelweed (*Impatiens* spp.). Crumble the long stock and rub it on poison ivy rash when it starts to itch. The itch fades slowly after each use, and each time it returns, the affected area will be smaller. The rash will completely disappear after a few good rubdowns.

Jewelweed

Apply a jewelweed poultice (*Impatiens* spp.) to cure poison ivy.

Jimson Weed

Apply the juice of jimson weed (*Datura stramonium*) directly to the rash. The stems provide the most juice, but the leaves also yield some.

Limewater, Salt

Treat poison ivy with limewater to which salt has been added.

Milkweed

Squeeze the milk from the broken off stems of milkweed (*Asclepias syriaca*) and apply to poison ivy rash.

> *It was like holding a match to it, but within an hour it had dried up. I have told a lot of people to use it, and they have with good results.* William E. Osborne

Nightshade

To stop the itch and eventually to cure poison ivy, make a lotion from several nightshade leaves (*Solanum nigrum*) by mashing them up in a teacup with the handle of a table knife. Add just a few drops of evaporated milk to the residue to make a pale green solution. Lightly rub or dab this on the ivy rash. It will stop the itching.

> *It works! Better than calamine!* Nelda Ellis

Nightshade

Crush nightshade leaves (*Solanum nigrum*) in a sauce dish and add just a little milk or cream. Use the mixture on the ivy infection.

A friend, then in her seventies, gave me this remedy forty years ago. Blanche Duzan

Nightshade

Wash and boil the leaves of nightshade (*Solanum nigrum*) in a small amount of water until tender. Add a few teaspoons of cornmeal to thicken the mixture. Spoon it onto a clean cotton cloth and fold it to contain the mixture. Apply to the affected area while warm and leave in place for 1 hour. The poultice is very effective for poison ivy.

Nightshade

Fry 6 or 8 nightshade leaves (*Solanum nigrum*) in butter for 5 minutes. Add 4 ounces of milk and heat gently for about 10 minutes. When cool, apply to poison ivy rash twice daily.

Poison Ivy

Eat poison ivy leaves (*Toxicodendron radicans*) to develop an immunity against the rash.

Pokeroot

Boil pokeroot (*Phytolacca americana*) in water to make an extract that is useful in treating poison ivy and other types of rashes as well.

I hope you try it out as it is so good for many rashes besides poison ivy. Mrs. Earl Wiles

Soap, Salt, Vinegar

To cure poison ivy rash, first wash with brown laundry soap. Then rub with a mixture of salt and vinegar.

Rubbed on hard this will cure the poison and leave a big scab. Madge Ellett

Sweet Spirit of Nitre

Bathe the affected area with sweet spirit of nitre 2 or 3 times during the day.

Next morning, scarcely any trace of the rash will remain. Sylvia P. Gibbons

White Shoe Polish

Apply white shoe polish to cure poison ivy rash.

Comments

More than 100 different plant juices have been reported in the literature as being used by the laity in the treatment of poison ivy. The number of such remedies reported by Hoosier informants therefore represents less than 10% of the possibilities. Nevertheless, the important ones are included in this listing, and of these, jewelweed is certainly the most significant and the most thoroughly studied. Based on the number of reports received, however, milkweed juice (latex) and the various nightshades are at least equal to jewelweed in popularity here in Indiana.

The scientific evidence regarding the value of jewelweed in treating rhus (poison ivy, poison sumac) dermatitis is conflicting. One study, in 1950, found it to be of no value. Another, reported by a physician in 1957, yielded favorable results. Of 115 patients treated, 108 were entirely relieved of their symptoms in two or three days. This investigator concluded that jewelweed is a very potent and safe therapeutic agent for the treatment of poison ivy dermatitis.

Nightshade leaves, usually mixed with a little milk or cream, are a highly respected remedy among Indiana informants for this troublesome condition; jimson weed also was often recommended, and one correspondent reported good results with deadly nightshade berries. Four different informants advocated milkweed as an effective remedy. Unfortunately, with a single exception, no critical scientific or medical studies regarding the effectiveness of these or any of the other remedies listed has been carried out.

The exception is the treatment involving eating poison ivy leaves themselves to develop an immunity to the rash. This is probably not very effective in most cases, but purified preparations of the toxin intended for oral use are currently marketed. If one does eat the leaves themselves, a practice I do not recommend, it is very important not to let them touch the skin surrounding the mouth. While the mucous membranes are not susceptible to poison ivy dermatitis, the skin around them certainly is.

Although there is little, if any, scientific evidence to support the effectiveness of many of the other suggested remedies, it should not be assumed that they are totally without value. Detergents (laundry soap), alkalis (limewater), and astringents (copperas, sugar of lead) may be modestly useful in removing any remaining toxin from the skin and in helping to allay the itching. White shoe polish with its content of zinc oxide or pipe clay would promote "drying" of the rash. The alcohol in the sweet spirit of nitre would have a similar effect.

⤳Rabies⤶

Elecampane

Take 1½ ounces of elecampane root (*Inula helenium*), powder or cut very fine, put it in a pint of fresh milk, and boil down to ½ pint. Take ⅓ of it in the early morning every other day until gone. Eat no food until 4:00 p.m. on those days. The remedy is an infallible treatment for hydrophobia if begun within 24 hours after the accident.

Pennyroyal

Pennyroyal tea (*Hedeoma pulegioides*) was used by the Indians to treat bites from rabid animals, if the bite was not higher than the shoulder. This was considered to be very important. The tea was drunk if the patient could swallow; otherwise it was applied as a wash. The wound was also packed with bruised fresh leaves or soaked dry leaves.

Comments

Neither of these remedies would be of any value in the treatment of rabies (hydrophobia). If they even appeared effective, it could only mean that either the animal inflicting the bite was not rabid or its teeth did not penetrate the skin of the victim.

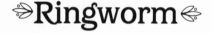

Ringworm

Black Walnut

Squeeze the juice from black walnut hulls (*Juglans nigra*) directly on a ringworm infection, and rub it in. The juice will heal the infection in a few days. For best results use walnuts that have fallen to the ground. The hulls are juicier.

Carrot

To cure ringworm, rub it with a carrot.

Cigar Ashes, Saliva

Moisten the ringworm infection with saliva and then rub cigar ashes thoroughly into the area. Repeat 3 times daily and it will be cured in a few days.

Milkweed

Ringworm can be cured by rubbing it with the milk from milk-weed stems (*Asclepias syriaca*). Apply daily for several days.

Pokeroot

A salve made by mixing lard with finely ground pokeroot or, alternatively, water in which pokeroots (*Phytolacca americana*) have been boiled is applied locally to cure ringworm.

Tobacco Dregs

Apply the tarry dregs from the bottom of a tobacco pipe to cure ringworm.

Tobacco Juice

For ringworm, apply tobacco juice (mixture of saliva and tobacco resulting from chewing tobacco).

Yellow Dock

A useful treatment for ringworm is prepared by soaking the leaves and stems of yellow dock (*Rumex crispus*) in vinegar. The liquid is simply applied to the affected areas and allowed to air dry.

Comments

Ringworm is a contagious disease of the skin, hair, or nails caused by several different kinds of fungi, all of which produce ring-shaped discolored patches on the skin, thus giving the condition its name. The remedies listed, with the notable exception of carrot, probably all have mild fungicidal properties and would therefore be somewhat effective.

Although it is a classical remedy for ringworm and the "itch" (scabies), pokeroot is a very poisonous herb. Even its external application, as noted here, cannot be recommended.

Scurvy

Watercress

Eat watercress (*Nasturtium officinale*) to cure or to prevent scurvy.

Comments

Scurvy is a vitamin-deficiency disease caused by a lack of vitamin C (ascorbic acid). That vitamin occurs abundantly in green leafy vegetables, so eating quantities of any of them would indeed prevent or cure the condition. Watercress contains about 25 milligrams of vitamin C per ounce.

Sexual Impotence

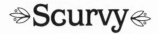

Ginseng

Take ginseng root (*Panax quinquefolius*) to improve sexual performance.

Narrow Dock

Narrow dock root, also known as yellow dock (*Rumex crispus*), is used as an aphrodisiac.

Comments

Narrow dock has a much greater reputation as an alterative, that is, a treatment for venereal disease, than it does as an aphrodisiac (an agent stimulating sexual desire and ability). Even its alterative reputation appears unfounded. About the best that can be said of narrow dock is that it has some laxative properties.

Ginseng is quite another matter. It has an age-old reputation in the Orient as a cure-all and, especially, as a sexual stimulant. In this country, it has become extremely popular as a so-called adaptogen, an agent that increases the body's resistance to disease by building up the general vitality and strengthening the normal body functions. As such, it might well be expected to have a beneficial effect on sexual activity. However, the Food and Drug Administration reported that it found no evidence that the use of ginseng enhanced sexual experience or potency. Can a billion Chinese be wrong?

⤳Skin Problems⤶ (Minor)

Burdock Root

Apply burdock root (*Arctium minus*) tea locally to cure acne.

Horseradish, Sour Milk

To remove freckles, grate some horseradish into very sour milk and let stand for 5 hours. Use this as a wash morning and night.

Lemon Juice

Apply lemon juice twice daily to make the skin fair or to remove freckles.

Milkweed

The complexion may be lightened and blemishes removed from the skin by applying milkweed milk (latex) (*Asclepius syriaca*), either pure or diluted with a little water.

Plantain Leaves

To relieve galling of the skin, apply plantain leaves (*Plantago* spp.) to the affected area.

Red Clover

Various skin irritations are relieved by the application of a clover poultice. Entire red clover plants (*Trifolium pratense*) are washed, cooked in a little water until tender, drained, and sprinkled with white flour. Place the mixture directly on the site and cover with a clean cotton cloth. Leave in place for several hours.

Rhubarb Stalk

To clean stains from under the fingernails, take a nice big rhubarb stalk (*Rheum rhaponticum*) and rub the fingernails right into it.

Starch

Use cornstarch as a dusting powder for prickly heat or diaper rash.

Stump Water

Water found standing in a hollow stump in the spring is a good treatment for a bad complexion.

Urine

To cure acne, drink your own urine.

Watermelon Juice

Complexion problems are remedied by bathing the skin in watermelon juice.

Wild Daisy

A useful remedy for diaper rash or chafing of the skin is prepared from wild daisy flowers (*Chrysanthemum leucanthemum*). Remove the yellow centers from flower heads and pulverize them in a mortar and pestle or by rubbing between two stones. Mix with melted lard, cook, and apply to the affected area.

Witch Hazel

To relieve skin redness (not rashes or burns), boil the leaves of witch hazel together with a little bit of the bark (*Hamamelis virginiana*) in water. Apply the extract to the inflammed area with a clean white cloth, then saturate the cloth and place it over the area until it dries out.

Comments

The skin problems considered here and the remedies suggested for them are quite varied. Horseradish in sour milk, lemon juice, and rhubarb stalk are employed for their acidic bleaching action. The oxalic acid which occurs in abundance in rhubarb, for example, is a very effective stain remover. The lactic acid in sour milk and the citric acid in lemon function in the same way.

Cornstarch forms a protective, absorbent layer on the skin. Burdock root contains the carbohydrate inulin with similar properties, and in addition, the fresh root may have some bacteriostatic effect. Watermelon juice and milkweed milk (latex) both tend to form protective coatings on drying.

Witch hazel leaves are rich in tannin and are a very useful astringent. The water standing in at least certain kinds of old stumps would probably also be a good source of astringent tannins, having leached them from the cells of its natural reservoir. Leaves of the familiar plantain are also useful, apparently due to their mucilaginous character, although in Europe antibiotic properties are also attributed to them.

Poultices and ointments or salves are both soothing in nature. They are thus beneficial for minor skin problems.

Drinking urine, even one's own, is not a healthful practice. It is not recommended.

⇒Slivers and Splinters⇐

Cheese Plant

An infection caused by a thorn or sliver is effectively treated by bathing the affected part with a hot solution made by boiling cheese plant (*Malva* spp.) in water.

Crabgrass, Bacon, Salt

Draw out splinters with a poultice made by moistening a large handful of crabgrass (*Digitaria sanguinalis*) with hot water until wilted. Drain, and mix with 1 tablespoonful of bacon drippings and ½ cup of salt. Put in a clean cloth and apply locally, leaving in place for several hours.

Olive Oil

Pat the area surrounding a splinter with a little olive oil and it will slip out easily.

Rosin

Even the deepest slivers may be removed by melting a little rosin on a piece of gauze and bandaging it over the affected area for 2 or 3 days.

Sugar, Soap

To remove a splinter, mix brown sugar with brown laundry soap and apply to the affected area. By the next day, the splinter will be drawn out.

Comments

Agents that soften and lubricate the tissue around the embedded particle or that otherwise exert a kind of "drawing" or astringent action are obviously beneficial in the removal of slivers, splinters, thorns, and similar objects from the skin. Bathing the area with hot water containing some mucilaginous plant material (cheese plant) or applying olive oil would function in the former manner. Rosin would act primarily as an astringent. Sugar and soap or the crabgrass, bacon, and salt poultice would tend to combine both softening and "drawing" effects.

⇘Snakebite⇖

Chewing Tobacco

A moist wad of chewing tobacco applied to the spot is a good treatment for snakebite.

Goldenseal Leaves

Put 2 pounds of goldenseal leaves (*Hydrastis canadensis*) in ½ gallon of vinegar and boil the liquid down to ½ pint. Take ½ to 1 tablespoonful 3 times daily.

Plantain

Drink the fresh juice from green plantain leaves (*Plantago* spp.) and apply the leaves externally to the punctures to cure rattlesnake bite.

Rattlesnake Master

The root of rattlesnake master (*Liatris* or *Agave* spp.) is an excellent remedy for snakebite. Boil it in milk and drink the mixture. The leaves of the plant can be made into a poultice that is also helpful when applied directly to the bite.

Snakeroot

Snakeroot (*Asarum, Aristolochia,* or *Eryngium* spp.) is used to cure snakebite.

Snakeweed

Chew the leaves of snakeweed (*Aristolochia serpentaria*) to cure snakebite.

Whiskey

Drink whiskey to cure snakebite.

Comments

None of these remedies is of any benefit whatsoever in the treatment of bites by poisonous snakes. As a matter of fact, they would be of minimum value in treating any kind of snakebite. Drinking whiskey would actually increase the danger from the bite of a poisonous snake. The alcohol would dilate the blood vessels and increase the victim's heart rate, thereby hastening the spread of the venom throughout the body.

Most of the remedies for snakebite are based on the long-discredited doctrine of signatures. Some part of the plant, usually the root, resembles a snake in appearance and is, therefore, assumed to be useful in treating the bite of the reptile.

⇒Sore Mouth⇐ (Canker Sores)

Potassium Chlorate

Canker sores in the mouth may be cured by gargling with warm potassium chlorate solution (1 teaspoonful in 1 cup of water).

Yellow Root

Rinse with yellow root tea (*Hydrastis canadensis*) to relieve a sore mouth.

Yellow Root

Yellow root tea (*Hydrastis canadenis*) cures sore mouth and cracked and bleeding lips.

> *I had a very sore mouth for about three years. All standard medical treatments failed. A friend told me about yellow root tea, and I used it regularly. In two weeks, my mouth was well. I have a lot of praise for yellow root.* Mrs. Wayne Hollen

Yellow Root

Dig yellow root (*Hydrastis canadensis*), scrape, and then chew it for canker sores in the mouth.

> *It is bitter, but it heals.* Mildred Dively

Comments

Yellow root, also commonly referred to as goldenseal or hydrastis, was so frequently and so enthusiastically recommended by informants as a cure for sore mouth and related problems that several variations of its use are listed here. The herb contains alkaloids that do have both astringent and weak antiseptic properties, so it probably is an effective treatment for many cases of sore mouth (stomatitis), canker sores, and the like.

Potassium chlorate is a feeble antiseptic. It is nevertheless used as a gargle in treating various inflammatory conditions of the mucous membranes of the mouth.

⇒Sores⇐

Black Walnut Hulls

Squeezing the juice from black walnut hulls (*Juglans nigra*) on the sore will heal it.

> *It burns like heck, but does the job.* James "Luke" Mann

Dog Saliva

"Summer sores" will heal rapidly after they have been licked thoroughly by a dog.

> *One of the most miraculous cures I have experienced.* Madge Ellett

Fat Meat; Salt Pork

Put a piece of fat meat or salt pork on the sore to draw out the poison.

Pokeroot

For running ulcers or sores, make a salve by boiling pokeroot (*Phytolacca americana*) until a strong extract is formed. Then thicken to a salve with flour, honey, eggs, and olive oil. Apply freely.

Turpentine

Turpentine treatment for open sores: put lard around the sore, then pour turpentine oil directly in it.

> *It is painful but reliable.* Mildred Dively

Comments

Sores are commonly associated with some kind of infection, so appropriate treatment involves application of a product with an antiseptic action. Black walnut hulls, with their content of quinones, fall in this category. They would, however, be a most unsightly treatment due to the nearly indelible stains which they produce on the skin.

Animals, including dogs, lick their own sores and wounds to help them heal. Their saliva undoubtedly possesses antiseptic properties. Note that dog saliva was previously reported as a cure for athlete's foot. The salt in salt pork could be beneficial, and turpentine oil not only is antiseptic but would also stimulate circulation around the sore through its counterirritant properties and thus promote healing. As noted by the correspondent, it would be quite painful if applied to an open sore.

Pokeroot in various forms has been recommended by our informants for all kinds of skin conditions including running ulcers or sores. Again, because of its toxicity, its use seems inadvisable.

⇘Sore Throat⇙

Black Pepper, Fat Meat

For a sore throat, sprinkle pepper on sliced fat meat and tie with a cloth around the throat.

> *I've always had sore throats, and I wore that*
> *all the time when I was small.* Thelma B. Fox

Cocklebur

A soothing remedy for sore throat is prepared from the leaves and roots of cocklebur (*Xanthium* spp.). Gather these plant parts and chop very fine or pulverize. Mix with a few teaspoonfuls of white flour and water. Place ½ teaspoonful on the back of the tongue and allow to drain into the throat. It is very effective.

Cranesbill

A mild tea made from cranesbill or wild geranium root (*Geranium maculatum*) will relieve sore throat. Drink ½ to 1 cupful every few hours.

Egg White, Lemon, Sugar

Relieve hoarseness by using the white of an egg, thoroughly beaten, mixed with lemon juice and sugar. Take a teaspoonful occasionally.

Flaxseed

For hoarseness or sore throat associated with a cold, apply a flaxseed poultice to the throat.

Horehound

Horehound tea (*Marrubium vulgare*) made into a syrup with honey is the standard Indiana remedy for sore throat.

Horseradish, Vinegar, Honey

To get rid of hoarseness, boil fresh horseradish root with cider vinegar and add some honey. Take as needed.

Lemon, Salt

For hoarseness, suck a lemon on which salt has been sprinkled.

Lovage

For tonsillitis, cut up lovage root (*Levisticum officinale*) and fry in lard. Apply externally to the throat as a poultice.

Mayweed

For a sore throat, make a mayweed (*Anthemis cotula*) poultice by bruising the plant to a soft pulp, boiling in a little water, thickening with cornmeal, and spreading on a thick cloth. Apply the poultice to the neck.

Sage

Drink sage tea (*Salvia officinalis*) to relieve a sore throat.

Salt Water

Soreness of the throat is relieved by simply gargling with warm salt water.

Sassafras

Drink sassafras tea (*Sassafras albidum*) to cure a sore throat.

Slippery Elm

Drink tea made from slippery elm bark (*Ulmus fulva*) to ease a sore throat.

Slippery Elm

Gargle with warm tea made from slippery elm bark (*Ulmus fulva*) to relieve a sore throat.

This is very good. Dorris B. Layman

Slippery Elm

Chew slippery elm bark (*Ulmus fulva*) vigorously to relieve a sore throat.

Smoked Side Meat

For sore throat, place a piece of smoked side meat over the affected area and cover with woolen cloth.

Spruce Cones

To soothe a sore throat, chew the tiny young cones of spruce trees (*Picea* spp.).

Sugar, Butter

Eat a mixture of sugar and butter to help a sore throat.

Turpentine, Kerosene, Lard

For sore throat, rub on a mixture of turpentine oil, kerosene, and lard.

> *That ought to chase anything away.* Irene Lankford

Vinegar, Salt Water

For a sore throat, gargle with vinegar and salt water.

Vinegar, Salt, Red Pepper, Alum

To relieve a sore throat, gargle with a mixture prepared from one teacup of vinegar, salt, red pepper (as strong as can be taken), and a bit of powdered alum. Use frequently.

Yellow Root

Take a teaspoonful of powdered yellow root (*Hydrastis canadensis*) in a glass of water to relieve sore throat.

Comments

Many of the remedies for sore throat are similar or identical to the recipes submitted for Colds and Flu or Coughs and Croup which have been previously listed and discussed under those headings. Here, too, we find antiseptics, aromatics, astringents, demulcents, and expectorants, as well as products or formulas combining several of these properties. Because of its volatile oil and tannin content, sage, for example, is an aromatic, an antiseptic, and an astringent. The same properties are found in the recipe recommending vinegar, salt, red pepper, and alum.

Cranesbill and yellow root are primarily astringents, horehound an expectorant, slippery elm and sugar and butter are demulcents, warm salt water an antiseptic, and so on. Most of the remedies are probably at least modestly effective. Nature usually cures a sore throat in a few days anyway, and unless one is using powerful antibacterial agents such as the antibiotics, the most that can be expected from any treatment is temporary relief.

⇨Sprains and Sore Muscles⇦

Angleworm Oil

The oil resulting when common angleworms are placed in a glass jar out in the sun and allowed to "melt" is an excellent liniment for sprains, muscular aches, and sore joints.

Arnica Flowers

Soak arnica flowers (*Arnica* spp.) in rubbing alcohol to prepare a liniment that is very effective for treating sore muscles and aching backs.

Balsam Pear, Camphor, Wintergreen

Place a balsam pear (*Momordica charantia*) in a jar and cover with rubbing alcohol in which have been dissolved about a tablespoonful of gum camphor and 2 tablespoonfuls of wintergreen oil. After a time, the fruits lose their bright orange color, and the brilliant red pulp in which the seeds are encased also loses its color. The liquid that is filtered off then makes a pleasant rub for sore and aching muscles.

> *I heard the pioneers made this with good bourbon whiskey, when it was less expensive, instead of rubbing alcohol. It was said to be a cure-all, drunk for internal ailments and rubbed on for external ones.* Helen Patrick

Compare this formula with Grandma's Arthritis Liniment (Balsam Cucumber, Witch Hazel, Wintergreen) in the section Arthritis and Rheumatism.

Boneset, Smartweed

For sprains, take equal parts of boneset herb *Eupatorium perfoliatum*) and smartweed (*Polygonum punctatum*) and soak in rubbing alcohol for 4 hours. Strain and bottle. Bathe the skin over the sprain freely with this liquid.

Epsom Salts

Soak in epsom salts and hot water to reduce the swelling associated with a sprain.

Kerosene

To relieve muscle cramps, bathe the part in kerosene.

Mayweed

A useful liniment for sore muscles and sprains is made by soaking mayweed or dogfennel blossoms (*Anthemis cotula*) in alcohol. Use as a rub.

Mud, White Walnut Bark

Relieve the pain in sprains and sore joints with a mud-bark pack prepared as follows. Remove the top layer of soil from a well-drained area and dig some of the mud from underneath. Add a little water if necessary. Chop white walnut bark (*Juglans cinerea*) into fine particles and mix thoroughly with the mud. Apply to the painful area, elevate the affected part, if possible, and allow the pack to remain until it crumbles away. The pack may be applied hot after warming the ingredients in a pan, but it is also effective cold.

Mullein

To cure a sprain, cut several mullein stalks (*Verbascum thapsus*) into small pieces. Boil in a quart of cider vinegar and apply while hot.

Mustard

A mustard plaster useful in treating sprains or strained muscles is prepared from the leaves and stems of the mustard plant (*Brassica* spp.) which, after gathering, are washed, cut into small pieces, and ground or mashed into a pulp. Coat the skin of the affected area with lard or vaseline, then cover with this pulp and bind tightly with a bandage. Coating of the skin is essential, otherwise the mustard has a tendency to "burn" it. Leave the plaster on for several hours or overnight for best results.

Mustard

Backache is relieved by applying a mustard plaster.

Salt, Lard

Mix salt (not iodized) with lard to form a thick poultice that is spread on a cloth which is then applied to the sprain and wrapped with more cloth to keep it from running out.

> *I know it takes out all the swelling because I tried it on a neighbor boy who sprained his ankle and couldn't get his shoe on. By next morning he was wearing a shoe.* Josephine Hayes

Turpentine, Camphor, Sassafras

An effective liniment for sprains and strains is prepared from:

Turpentine oil	1 pint
Camphor spirit	1 pint
Sassafras oil	½ ounce
Olive oil	a small amount
Mix and rub on as needed.	

> *It is effective for horses and humans.* John Edward Hopkins

Turpentine, Vinegar, Eggs

Liniment for sprains, sore muscles, etc.:

Turpentine oil	½ pint
White vinegar	1 pint
Fresh eggs	2

Put the turpentine oil in a glass jar. Break the eggs in a cup and beat them. Then put the eggs and the shells in the turpentine oil and add the vinegar. Let it stand in the jar (sealed) a day or two. Shake before using.

Urine

For a sore and swollen knee, soak a cloth in your own urine and wrap it around the joint.

Vinegar

For a sprain, add salt to cider vinegar, warm, and rub on.

Wormwood, Vinegar

For a sprain, rub on a liniment made by soaking bruised worm-wood stalks (*Artemesia absinthium*) in vinegar.

Wild Mint; Spikenard

Crush any of the wild mint plants (*Blephilia, Monarda,* or *Pycnanthemum* spp.) or spikenard root (*Aralia racemosa*) and mix with vegetable oil. Let it stand several days, strain, and use as a massage lotion for a sore back.

Comments

Sprains and sore muscles are usually treated by one or more of the following methods: 1. application of counterirritants or rubifacients, that is, agents which produce a degree of superficial irritation marked by locally increased blood flow to relieve the more severe irritation of a deeper-lying adjacent structure; 2. use of hot packs or soaking in hot water, both of which also increase the circulation of the blood in the area being treated; 3. rubbing or massage which performs much the same role.

Most liniments, unless they actually contain an analgesic, rely as much on the method of application, namely the rubbing in, for their effectiveness as on their actual composition. The balsam pear-camphor-wintergreen preparation listed is one of the exceptions because it contains methyl salicylate (wintergreen oil). This has an analgesic action similar to that of aspirin and also stimulates the flow of blood to the affected part when applied locally. In doing so, it reddens the skin and is thus said to act as a rubefacient. Arnica also contains compounds that have analgesic and anti-inflammatory properties.

Turpentine, vinegar, wormwood, sassafras, even wild mints, all act as counterirritants. Mustard plasters are a bit stronger, being rubifacients (causing reddening of the skin). As our correspondent notes, one must be careful in using them or they are liable to become vesicants (produce blistering). Epsom salts and hot water are effective primarily because of the high temperature of the water. The mud pack containing white walnut bark would be much more effective hot than cold.

⇒Sties⇐

Potato

To treat a sty, take fresh scrapings from the inside of an Irish potato, put them on a piece of clean cloth, and place on the sty. Replace once or twice with fresh scrapings.

> *This remedy was probably passed on to my mother by her parents who were born in the 1850s and '60s. It was amazingly effective. Within a couple of hours, the swelling was down, and the sty was significantly improved. By that evening, it was almost gone.* Judith Fehrmann

Comments

Sties are swollen, inflamed sebaceous glands on the margins of the eyelids. Most of the cures submitted for them, like those for warts, involved magic or superstition. This is the only one that did not. However, if it is effective in curing the causative infection, I am unable to explain why or how it works.

⇗Stomachache and Colic⇖

Bloodroot

Boil bloodroot (*Sanguinaria canadensis*) in water to make a strong solution. Strain, and drink up to ½ cupful to cure the colic.

Buttonweed

Drink buttonweed tea (*Diodia teres*) to cure a stomachache.

> *That was worse than a bellyache.* Earl York

Caraway; Anise; Dill

Chew caraway seeds (*Carum carvi*), anise seeds (*Pimpinella anisum*), or dill seeds (*Anethum graveolens*) to "ease" the stomach.

Castor Oil

To treat colic in infants, rub warm castor oil on the stomach and keep covered with warm cloths.

Castor Oil, Turpentine

A teaspoonful of turpentine oil mixed with a tablespoonful of castor oil is effective for colic or stomachache.

Catnip

Catnip tea (*Nepeta cataria*) is drunk to cure stomach upset or indigestion. It is also good to relieve colic in infants.

Chamomile

Drink chamomile tea (*Anthemis nobilis*) to ease an upset stomach.

Cinnamon

To relieve an upset stomach, take about ¼ teaspoonful of powdered cinnamon with a glass of water.

Comfrey

Comfrey leaf tea (*Symphytum officinale*) provides great relief for stomach ailments.

Crawley Root

Colic is relieved by drinking tea made from crawley root (*Corallorrhiza odontorhiza*), otherwise known as coralroot. It should be sweetened with honey.

Dandelion

To aid digestion, collect the small leaves of the dandelion plant (*Taraxacum officinale*). (The larger leaves are bitter.) Wash and place them in boiling water in a covered ceramic pot. Steep until the leaves are tender. Add a few mint leaves to flavor and sugar to taste. Sip a small cupful of the hot beverage after meals.

Dill

Dillseed tea (*Anethum graveolens*) will relieve the colic in infants and lull them to sleep.

Dogfennel

Make a tea from the yellow middle part of the flower of dogfennel (*Anthemis cotula*) and drink to cure an upset stomach.

Ginger Root

Tea prepared from ginger root is good for upset stomach.

Herbs (Various)

Colic in infants or children is treated with warm, sweetened teas made from any one of the following herbs or spices: catnip (*Nepeta cataria*), an Indiana favorite; peppermint (*Mentha piperita*); spearmint (*Mentha spicata*); pennyroyal (*Hedeoma pulegioides*); calamus roots (*Acorus calamus*); or cinnamon.

Horseradish

Place bruised horseradish leaves (*Armoracia rusticana*) directly on the skin over the stomach to cure aching.

Peach Tree Twigs

For an upset stomach, drink tea made by boiling the new growth (leaves and twigs) of a peach tree (*Prunus persica*) in water.

Pennyroyal

Pennyroyal tea (*Hedeoma pulegioides*) is useful in relieving colic.

Peppermint Oil, Sugar

Drink hot water to which sugar and peppermint oil have been added in order to calm an upset stomach.

Peppermint

Drink boiled peppermint tea (*Mentha piperita*) to cure a stomachache.

Peppermint; Spearmint

Drink peppermint (*Mentha piperita*) or spearmint (*Mentha spicata*) tea to relieve an upset stomach.

Spearmint

Chew spearmint leaves (*Mentha spicata*) to relieve a stomachache.

Sage

Drink sage tea (*Salvia officinalis*) for an upset stomach.

Salt Water

To relieve colic in an infant, administer a few drops of warm salt water.

Sheep Manure

Tea made from sheep droppings is good for all stomach troubles.

Sheep Sorrel, Wild Mint

To alleviate upset stomach and/or nausea, gather the leaves and stems of sheep sorrel (*Rumex acetosella*) and an equal quantity of wild mint (*Blephilia, Monarda,* or *Pycnanthemum* spp.) Wash and boil in a little water until the leaves are tender. Pour the water off and allow to cool until just warm. Take 3 or 4 tablespoons of the brew.

Summer Savory

Tea made from summer savory (*Satureja hortensis*) is good for an upset stomach.

Thyme

Thyme tea (*Thymus vulgaris*) is recommended for a stomachache.

Unicorn Root

A superior remedy for colic is unicorn or stargrass root (*Aletris farinosa*). It should be dug fresh, washed well, and made into a strong tea. Drink it several times daily to obtain relief.

Whiskey, Water, Sugar

For colic or stomachache in adults, drink whiskey mixed with warm water and sugar.

Wild Geranium

Tea made from wild geranium root (*Geranium maculatum*) is good for an upset stomach.

Wild Mint

Drink wild mint tea (*Blephilia, Monarda,* or *Pycnanthemum* spp.) to cure an upset stomach.

Wild Mint

To settle an upset stomach, collect wild mint plants (*Blephilia, Monarda,* or *Pycnanthemum* spp.), wash well, place in boiling water, and boil for 10 minutes. Remove from the heat, drain the liquid off, and discard the leaves. Add ½ cup of honey to the broth and store in bottles. Take 3 tablespoonfuls as needed.

Wild Onions; Wild Garlic

The fresh tops of wild onions and garlic (*Allium* spp.) collected in the early spring and lightly sauteed in butter are excellent aids to the digestion.

Yellow Root

Chew yellow root (*Hydrastis canadensis*) to relieve an upset stomach.

Yellow Root

Take a teaspoonful of yellow root (*Hydrastis canadensis*) in a glass of water for stomach troubles.

Comments

Most of the remedies in this category are carminatives, that is, agents that help expel gas and otherwise aid the digestive process. In this category are the various hot teas and similar preparations made from catnip, cinnamon, ginger, peppermint, sage, spearmint, summer savory, thyme, and wild mint, among others. Also included are the seeds (actually the fruits) of anise, caraway, and dill which, according to the correspondent, may be chewed.

Chamomile is a carminative, but it has, in addition, antispasmodic (relaxes smooth muscle) and anti-inflammatory properties. It is, therefore, a particularly valuable digestive aid.

In addition to its astringent properties, yellow root is very bitter and has long had the reputation of aiding digestion and helping various stomach problems. (See the section Stomach Ulcers.) Both garlic and onions are also said to provide relief from stomach ailments.

Castor oil, taken internally, is a powerful cathartic and would provide relief from stomachache due to constipation. Its action is quite vigorous, however, and it should not be used indiscriminately. Usually a milder laxative will serve.

Four other products mentioned are definitely not recommended. Sheep manure tea is not only unpalatable but also unsanitary. Bloodroot has been shown to be too toxic for human consumption. Calamus may aid digestion, but the volatile oil it contains has been shown to produce malignant tumors when fed to rats. Its consumption by humans is best avoided. Comfrey leaf also falls in this category. Having been shown to cause cancer of the liver in small animals, it should not be used internally.

⇒Stomach Ulcers ⇐

Flaxseed

Flaxseed is a sure cure for stomach ulcers. Take 1 teaspoonful of flaxseed and place it in a cup of water. Cover and let stand for 10 minutes. Then stir the mixture well and drink both water and flaxseed. Do this every night before going to bed for 2 or 3 months.

Garlic

To treat a stress-related ulcer, slice off a small piece of a clove of garlic and swallow it with a glass of water followed by breakfast.

Goldenrod

Make tea from the flowers, leaves, and stalk of common golden-rod (*Solidago* spp.) for stomach ulcers. Sip 3 or 4 cups a day, sweetened a little, to relieve the pain immediately. Collect and dry the plant in the late summer for year-round use.

> *This original recipe was given to me by Charles Elmer Fox who obtained it from the prairie Indians while he was a hobo during the depression. It is the best thing I ever used for severe stomach ulcers.* Sylvia Schwartz

Yellow Root

To cure a stomach ulcer, or any pain in the stomach, drink yellow root tea (*Hydrastis canadensis*).

Comments

Flaxseed contains large amounts of mucilage which expands in water and tends to coat the lining of the stomach and the ulcer, thereby preventing contact with the irritant acidic digestive juices.

As noted in the section Stomachache and Colic, garlic has a considerable reputation in the treatment of stomach disorders including ulcers. Indeed, scientists have been able to demonstrate its beneficial effects on such conditions in small animals. Unfortunately, the active principles responsible for such action have not been identified.

Goldenrod is noted in the literature as a carminative. There is nothing to explain its purported virtues for stomach ulcers.

The value of yellow root in various stomach conditions has, like that of garlic, been previously noted. Its helpful effects are thought to be primarily of an astringent nature.

⋙Thirst⋘

Chicory Root

Dry, roast, and grind chicory root (*Chicorium intybus*) to be used as a substitute for coffee.

Oswego Tea

Oswego tea (*Monarda didyma*) makes a very pleasant beverage and useful substitute for regular tea.

Sumac

The red velvet berries of sumac (*Rhus glabra*) can be used to make a very refreshing lemonade-type drink. The flavor is in the small hairs covering the berries. To prepare, soak a short time in cold water, strain through a piece of cloth to remove the hairs, and sweeten to taste.

Comments

Three pleasant, somewhat nonconventional beverages were reported by informants. Of the three products, only the chicory root is commonly used, being mixed with coffee to prepare the standard hot beverage of the New Orleans area.

❧Tobacco-Chewing Habit❧ (to Break)

Sassafras

Chew the root or stem bark of sassafras (*Sassafras albidum*) to break the tobacco-chewing habit.

Comments

Because of its pleasant taste, sassafras was no doubt once thought of as a pleasant substitute for chewing tobacco and considered helpful in weaning addicts from the untidy habit. Unfortunately, we now know that the herb contains large amounts of cancer-causing safrole. It would be imprudent to chew the bark for a prolonged period. It is, of course, also imprudent to chew cancer-causing tobacco. No one really knows which product is more harmful to use. It is certainly best to avoid both.

In Europe, the chewing of calamus rhizome (*Acorus calamus*) is frequently recommended as an aid in breaking the smoking habit. Since calamus contains β-asarone, a compound that, like the safrole in sassafras, has been found to cause cancer in animals, this practice, too, cannot be recommended. Nonetheless, it is interesting that, in both these cases, one cancer-causing product has been recommended as a means of overcoming habituation to another such material, specifically tobacco.

❧Tooth and Gum Problems❧

Alum

Apply powdered alum directly to relieve an aching tooth.

Ammonia

Saturate a bit of cotton with ammonia solution and apply to an aching tooth.

Baking Soda, Salt

Clean teeth with a mixture of baking soda and salt rubbed on with a rag.

Black Gum

Use twigs from the black gum tree (*Nyssa sylvatica*) as tooth-brushes.

>*They are free.* Sarah W. "Penny" Coleman

Bull Thistle

Chew the root of the bull thistle (*Cirsium vulgare*) to cure even the worst case of toothache.

Camphor

Rub camphor on the affected tooth and gum to relieve a tooth-ache.

Charcoal

To whiten teeth, rub them with powdered charcoal.

Clove Oil

Toothache is relieved by rubbing the affected tooth and gum with clove oil.

Fig

A fig is split open and applied as a poultice to cure a gum boil (abscess).

Garlic, Salt

To cure a toothache caused by a cavity, dip some garlic in salt and pack it in the hole. Then lie down on the side with the aching tooth, open your mouth, and let the garlic juice and saliva drip out. Your toothache will be gone.

> *I used this myself, and it really helped.* Rose Nisenbaum

Job's Tears

Hang a string of seeds of Job's tears (*Coix lachryma-jobi*) around the neck of a child to facilitate teething. When fresh, the seeds are soft and may be strung easily. They then become slick and bright and hard.

Northern Prickly Ash

Pack dried root bark from the toothache tree or northern prickly ash (*Zanthoxylum americanum*) in the cavity 2 or 3 times daily to relieve an aching tooth.

Nutmeg

A nutmeg poultice applied to the jaw will reduce the swelling around abscessed teeth.

Peppermint, Nettle

A good toothache remedy is prepared from the leaves of the wild peppermint (*Mentha piperita*) and from the roots of the prickly nettle (*Urtica* spp.). Collect equal amounts of these plant parts, wash thoroughly, mix, and chew well. Then surround the tooth, or pack the cavity, with the chewed quid. Allow to remain for about 1 hour.

and Yarrow

If ache persists, take fresh yarrow leaves (*Achillea millefolium*), wash, chew, and pack around the tooth as before. Allow this to remain for about ½ hour to obtain additional relief.

Raisin

Place a raisin in the cavity to stop a toothache.

Sassafras

To heal sore gums, cut a tender sassafras (*Sassafras albidum*) branch that is about the thickness of a pencil. Using a sharp knife, cut the ends of the branch lengthwise repeatedly to a depth of about ½ inch until they become somewhat frayed. Use like a toothbrush, being sure to cover the areas where tooth and gum meet. It will also whiten the teeth.

Slippery Elm Bark

Inflammation of the jaw caused by an aching tooth is relieved with a slippery elm bark (*Ulmus fulva*) poultice.

Sour Dock

The fried and powdered root of a sour dock (*Rumex crispus*) is used as a dentifrice.

Tobacco

Hold a wad of chewing tobacco on the tooth for toothache.

Comments

Any suitably abrasive material may be used to clean the teeth. The mixture of baking soda and salt is an old standby, and if you do not have a toothbrush, rub it on with a rag. Charcoal and powdered sour dock (yellow dock) root are similarly useful products.

Cleaning sticks of the types described under sassafras and black gum are probably used by more people around the world than are toothbrushes. Learned essays have been written, listing and describing the various varieties and the species of plants from which they are obtained. Personally, I would prefer not to used a sassafras stick, at least habitually, but it probably would not be too serious a matter if the bark was removed.

Anything relatively hard that a teething child bites down on will naturally facilitate penetration of the teeth through the gums. The seeds of Job's tears fall in this category. String them in such a way that the child cannot swallow them.

Many materials, particularly those containing certain volatile oils, have a useful local anesthetic action when applied to an aching tooth or, particularly, when packed into the cavity of such a tooth. The best is clove oil, but some of the other remedies listed may work, too. A relatively innocuous product, like the raisin, would probably function only if the ache were caused by air reaching an exposed nerve in the cavity; it could not possibly serve any role other than that of a mechanical plug or block.

✥Tuberculosis✥

Aloe

Cook aloe vera leaves (*Aloe barbadensis*) in water and honey to prepare a syrup that is a very effective treatment for tuberculosis. Take about 3 or 4 teaspoonfuls a day.

> *My mother prepared a constant supply of this for a cousin who was hospitalized in a TB sanatorium. The doctors could not understand how she healed so quickly. Today, she is in her eighties and still living.* Lillian N. Rosner

Black Nightshade

Tea prepared from the leaves of black nightshade (*Solanum nigrum*) is an old Indian remedy for tuberculosis.

Devil's Tongue

Boil devil's tongue leaves (*Sansevieria* spp.) in water and drink the resulting beverage for tuberculosis.

Elderberries

To treat tuberculosis, simmer down the juice of fresh elderberries (*Sambucus canadensis*) to a molasses-like consistency and add a little sugar. Take 1 teaspoonful 3 times daily mixed with ½ teaspoonful of fresh butter or olive oil. This will strengthen the lungs, heal the ulcers, ease the cough, and keep the bowels in a proper state.

Herbal Mixture

To cure tuberculosis, boil a handful each of horehound (*Marrubium vulgare*), spikenard (*Aralia racemosa*), and elecampane (*Inula helenium*) in water. Add ½ pint of honey and a large quantity of alum. Take 1 tablespoonful 3 times a day.

Herbal Mixture

For consumption (tuberculosis), add a little unslaked lime (calcium oxide) to 1 gallon of water. Hang in the water a cloth bag containing leaves of ground ivy (*Glechoma hederacea*), powdered horehound roots (*Marrubium vulgare*), powdered sweet anise seeds (*Osmorhiza longistylis*), and 1 tablespoonful of rosin. Take 3 tablespoonfuls a day of the extract stirred in a little milk.

Hops

For tuberculosis, take a cupful of finely powdered hops (*Humulus* spp.) and put it in a quart of good rye whiskey. Take 2 tablespoonfuls in the morning, 1 at noon, 1 in the evening, and 2 before going to bed.

Horehound, Mullein, Molasses

Mix 1 cup of strong horehound tea (*Marrubium vulgare*) with 1 cup of strong mullein leaf tea (*Verbascum thapsus*). Add 1 cupful of molasses and quickly boil to a syrup. Take a large swallow 3 times daily. It will cure all cases of tuberculosis that are not too far advanced.

Horse Manure

To cure tuberculosis, spread horse manure liberally all around the outside of the house where you live, and you will soon get well.

Peppermint

Soak peppermint (*Mentha piperita*) leaves in water, add a little sugar, and drink frequently to cure tuberculosis.

Pokeberries

Have the patient drink pokeberry juice (*Phytolacca americana*) to cure tuberculosis.

Comments

In spite of the enthusiastic endorsement of some of the submitted recipes by their contributors, none of them will cure tuberculosis. It would be folly to utilize any of these home remedies instead of seeking competent medical treatment.

⇒Warts⇐

Bacon (Pork) Rind

Put on a piece of bacon rind or pork rind to remove a wart.

Castor Oil

Rub castor oil on a wart morning and night. It will soon disappear.

Castor Oil, Sulfur

A mixture of castor oil and sulfur, applied frequently, will remove a wart.

Grasshopper Spittle

Apply grasshopper spittle to remove warts.

Milkweed

Milkweed milk (latex) (*Asclepias syriaca*) is an effective wart remover. Apply daily for several days until the wart goes away.

Milkweed

To remove a wart, first soak it in warm water. Then, using a needle sterilzed in flame, make several holes around the base of the wart. Finally, apply the milk (latex) from milkweed (*Asclepias syriaca*).

Potato

Split a potato and rub the freshly cut portion on the wart. It will disappear after 7 or 8 treatments.

Potato Water

To cure warts on the hands, boil potatoes in a little water and wash your hands in the juice.

Snail

Rub a snail on a wart to make it disappear.

Stump Water

To remove warts, dip them twice a day in water standing in an old, partially decayed, hollow stump.

Willow Ashes

The ashes of the common willow (*Salix* spp.) are mixed with cider vinegar and applied locally to remove warts.

This is more effective than milkweed juice. Mrs. Parker Layman

Comments

Many persons believe that psychic processes play a significant role in the removal of warts. Consequently, most of the wart cures submitted by Hoosier informants were more magical than medicinal. The few that were not, or apparently not, based primarily on superstition are listed here. Of these, the most popular is certainly milkweed milk or latex which was recommended by several different correspondents. Effective or not, it is at least widely known and used.

The magical cures not included here often involve subsequent burial of the object (potato, bacon rind, etc.) that has been rubbed on to make the wart disappear. A cure does not occur until the material rots in the ground. Some of the remedies reported may simply be shortened versions of this procedure.

Everyone who has read *Tom Sawyer* is familiar with spunk (stump) water as a wart cure. In spite of its probably purely magical significance, it is included here for two reasons. One is that it seems no less likely a potential cure than most of the others, potato water, for example. The other reason is that water that has stood for some time in stumps, especially oak stumps as are often suggested in connection with this remedy, may contain tannins and other dissolved materials that do have some beneficial effects on warts. No one really knows.

⇒Whooping Cough⇐

Chestnut Leaves

Boil chestnut leaves (*Castanea dentata*) in water and add sugar to make a syrup for the treatment of whooping cough.

Clover Blossoms

Tea made from clover blossoms (*Trifolium* spp.) will cure the whooping cough.

White Ants

Tea made from white ants will cure whooping cough.

Comments

The organisms that cause whooping cough or pertussis irritate the trachea or windpipe resulting in a convulsive, spasmodic cough. Methods of overcoming such irritations are discussed in general in the section Coughs and Croup. Three remedies recommended specifically for whooping cough are listed here.

⇒Worms⇐

Blue Flag

The juice of the blue flag plant (*Iris* spp.) is used to expel tapeworms.

Butternut Bark

For worms in children, give a syrup made by boiling butternut bark (*Juglans cinerea*) in water and adding about ⅓ the volume of molasses plus a little whiskey.

Potatoes

Eat raw potatoes to cure pinworms.

Pumpkin Seeds

Eat the kernels from the pumpkin seeds to cure worms.

Salt Herring, Pumpkin Seeds

To cure tapeworms, eat salt herring without drinking any water and follow with a quantity of pumpkin seeds.

Sauerkraut

Eat lots of raw sauerkraut to get rid of worms.

Spearmint

Make a tea by steeping ½ ounce of spearmint (*Mentha spicata*) in 1 pint of hot water for 15 minutes. Strain and drink to expel worms.

Sugar, Kerosene

Worms are expelled by eating a heaping teaspoonful of sugar to which a few drops of kerosene have been added.

Sugar, Turpentine

For worms, mix 8 or 9 drops of turpentine oil with a spoonful of sugar and eat it. Use periodically to keep from getting worms.

Tobacco Seed

Take tobacco seeds (*Nicotiana tabacum*) in molasses to cure worms.

Wormroot

To get rid of worms, drink wormroot tea (*Spigelia marilandica*).

Wormseed

The seeds of wormseed, or as it is commonly called in Indiana, vermifuge (*Chenopodium ambrosioides*), are taken to expel worms.

Comments

Many of the submitted remedies do act as anthelmintics or vermifuges, that is, they expel or otherwise destroy intestinal worms. Agents known to be effective when administered in proper quantities include blue flag, butternut bark, pumpkin seeds, turpentine oil, and wormroot. Both kerosene and tobacco seeds might also be effective, but they are really too toxic to be used internally in the necessary amounts.

One source identified spearmint tea as a powerful vermifuge, but there is nothing in the literature to confirm its effectiveness. It is also difficult to attribute much activity to raw potatoes or even to quantities of sauerkraut. These remedies are probably more fanciful than real.

❧Wounds❧

Bread, Milk

Wounds or festering sores are treated with a poultice of bread soaked in milk. Apply and keep wet with milk.

Bread, Tea

A bread and tea poultice applied to a wound will prevent blood poisoning (tetanus).

Chewing Tobacco

Apply a moist wad of chewing tobacco as a poultice to cure a puncture wound.

Comfrey

Comfrey poultice for wounds: chop up or blend 6 or more large comfrey leaves (*Symphytum officinale*), apply to wound, and wrap with a bandage. Save the juice and use to moisten bandage when dried out. Change every 24 hours. The treatment is also good for boils.

Cow Manure

To prevent infection after stepping on a rusty nail, apply a cow manure poultice to the injury.

Dirt

Dirt applied in or around a wound will keep away infection.

Ear Wax

If pierced ears fail to heal properly, rub wax from your ear on the bars of the ear rings and they will heal overnight.

Heal-All

Mix finely chopped heal-all (*Prunella vulgaris*) with lard to make a salve for treating wounds and cuts.

Kerosene

Apply kerosene to a deep wound caused by a nail or by barbed wire. It will stop the bleeding and prevent lockjaw.

Laundry Soap

Apply laundry soap to heal wounds.

Laundry Soap, Sugar

Laundry soap and sugar will heal wounds.

Laundry Soap, Sugar, Turpentine

Wash a severe wound thoroughly with laundry soap. Put on sugar and turpentine oil and bandage tightly. Do not change bandage too often, but pour more turpentine on daily. When bandage is changed, add more sugar.

Moldy Bread

Put moldy bread on an infected wound or abscess.

Onions

Eat large quantities of onions to eliminate any kind of infection in the body.

Onions

Apply slightly sauteed onions as a poultice for minor infections.

Peach Tree Leaves

To cure an infected wound or cut, pick a "bunch" of leaves from a peach tree (*Prunus persica*) and boil them in water until it turns dark. Soak the infected part in this liquid, just as hot as you can stand, 3 times a day.

> *This original recipe came from a neighbor lady, Peach Sterrett, who was wise in the ways of herbal medicine. I had blood poisoning from a cut on my toe. After a few days of this treatment, my foot was completely well.* Edna S. Northerner

Peach Tree Leaves

Bruise peach tree leaves (*Prunus persica*), apply them to the wounds, and bandage. Do this twice daily.

> *This will give quick relief; the pain will leave almost at once.* Ruby Dawson

Plantain Leaves

For puncture wounds or cuts caused by rusty metal and therefore subject to blood poisoning (tetanus), collect plantain leaves (*Plantago* spp.), wash and place in a clean white cloth. Place on a clean wooden block and hammer them to a pulp. Apply directly to the injured part.

Red Alder

Apply a poultice made of red alder bark (*Alnus* spp.) to cure infected wounds.

Salt Pork, Turpentine

To draw the infection from a wound, put salt pork and turpentine oil on it.

Slippery Elm, Rosin, Carbolic Acid

A useful ointment for infected wounds is made by boiling a large handful of slippery elm bark (*Ulmus fulva*) in water until it gets thick and slippery. Remove the pieces of bark, add 1 cup of lard, ½ cup of tallow, and a piece of rosin the size of a hulled walnut. Boil down until the water has disappeared and add a few drops of carbolic acid.

> *This has been known to cure wounds when doctors have failed.* Eva Brandt

Smartweed

For a foot wound made by a rusty nail, collect a bunch of smartweed (*Polygonum punctatum*) that is about knee high and cover with boiling water and continue boiling until it turns a brownish color. While the water is still very hot, soak the foot in it.

Spikenard

To treat blood poisoning (tetanus) in a puncture wound, boil spignet or spikenard root (*Aralia racemosa*) until soft, mash thoroughly, and make into a poultice which is applied directly to the wound.

> *By the next morning, all of the swelling was gone from a foot that had been badly infected.*
> Irene Lankford

Sulfur, Lard

Mix sulfur with lard and apply to infected wounds.

Comments

Most of the comments made in the section Cuts, Bruises, and Abrasions also apply here and to the next section, Wounds (Mixed) as well. Previous remarks made in the section Burns (Sunburn), and in the section Sprains and Sore Muscles, are pertinent to remedies listed in the next section. All of these prior comments will not be repeated other than to note the interesting recurrence of plantain leaves, peach tree leaves, and onions as well, for the treatment of infected wounds, even those of the puncture type which are so subject to lockjaw (tetanus).

The remedies, in general, possess antiseptic, styptic, and demulcent or protective properties. Moldy bread is often pointed out as a forerunner of penicillin or similar antibiotics produced by fungi. This always seemed to me to be somewhat farfetched. Most wild strains of mold produce very small amounts indeed of antibiotics.

It is wise not to rely too much on the remedies suggested for treatment of the puncture wounds. They may be alright if your tetanus shots are up-to-date; otherwise, consult a physician if you step on a rusty nail in the barnyard.

It is extremely unwise to apply dirt to any wound purposely. That measure recommended by one informant should certainly not be utilized. Although the soil is the richest source of microorganisms capable of producing useful antibiotics, it is also a source of pathogenic organisms that cause serious infections, e.g., tetanus or typhoid fever, in humans.

I tried not to include many recipes that would probably have to be compounded by a pharmacist, but I did list the phenol, glycerin, rose water, and bay rum recipe in the next section. The correspondent noted that it was so useful for so many different external ailments that I just could not resist. Maybe you, too, will find it useful.

➷Wounds, Cuts, Burns, Sprains, Sores, etc. ⤶ (Mixed)

Aloe Juice

The fresh juice of the aloe vera plant (*Aloe barbadensis*) is a useful treatment for minor cuts and burns. It is also useful for cuts and abrasions on dogs.

Balm of Gilead Buds

A useful balm of Gilead preparation (*Populus candicans*) is a tincture made by filling a small bottle ¼ full with the buds and then filling the rest of the way with rubbing alcohol or vodka. Let stand 1 week. It is an excellent remedy for application to cuts, bruises, or raw sores.

Castor Oil

To facilitate the healing of cuts, sores, or abrasions, use a feather to apply a little castor oil.

Egg White, Salt

The white of an egg and salt, mixed to thick paste, is one of the best remedies for sprains, bruises, or lameness in man or beast. Simply rub it well on the part affected.

Horseradish Leaves

Fresh horseradish leaves (*Armoracia rusticana*) are wet with vinegar and applied locally to sprains, bruises, cuts, abrasions, and the like.

Peach Tree Leaves

For bruises or burns, apply peach tree leaves (*Prunus persica*) to the skin, smooth side down. Bind them on with a cloth.

Phenol, Glycerin, Rose Water, Bay Rum

A simple, compounded remedy that is very effective for burns, cuts, cold sores, frostbite, dandruff, etc. is:

Phenol	4 drams
Glycerin	2 fluid ounces
Rose Water	6 fluid ounces
Bay Rum	8 fluid ounces

Rosin, Lard, Beeswax

An effective salve for cuts, and burns is prepared by melting and mixing ½ pound of lard with ¼ pound of beeswax and ¼ pound of rosin. Apply to the wound on a soft cotton cloth.

Sour Apple

To treat burns or wounds that are liable to become infected, apply apple salve prepared as follows: Fry a large, sliced but unpeeled, sour apple in a cup of lard. Add a piece of beeswax the size of a hulled walnut. When the wax is melted, strain the liquid into a jar that can be covered with a lid. Apply as necessary.

Turpentine, Cider Vinegar, Egg

Sprains, bruises, and cuts are treated with a liniment made from 1 egg beaten lightly, ½ pint of turpentine spirits, and ½ pint of apple cider vinegar. Shake well before using.

White Easter Lily

An ointment made from the leaves of the white Easter lily (*Lilium longiflorum*) and melted beeswax is very effective for the treatment of all minor injuries.

> *This is my Grandma Brown's famous White Lily Salve.* Ola B. Chillson

Comments

Most of the remarks in the section Cuts, Bruises, and Abrasions, in the section Burns (Sunburn), and in the section Sprains and Sore Muscles are pertinent to remedies listed here. See the explanation in the section Wounds.

Appendix
Botanical Names
Common and Scientific

A

Alder—*See* Swamp alder for a listing of the two species native to Indiana.

Alfalfa—*Medicago sativa* L.

Aloe—*Aloe barbadensis* Mill. = *Aloe vera* (L.) Webb & Berth.

Aloe vera—*See* Aloe.

Alum Root—In Indiana, this usually refers to *Heuchera americana* var. *brevipetala* Rosendahl, Butters, & Lakela; it is sometimes applied to *Geranium maculatum* L. as well. The roots of both plants are highly astringent.

American centaury—*Sabatia angularis* (L.) Pursh.

Anise—*Piminella anisum* L.

Arnica—European arnica derives from *Arnica montana* L.; American species, none of which is native to Indiana, include *Arnica fulgens* Pursh, *Arnica sororia* Greene, and *Arnica cordifolia* Hook.

Asafetida—*Ferula assafoetida* L. and related species.

B

Balm—*Melissa officinalis* L.

Balm of Gilead—*Populus candicans* Ait. = *Populus balsamifera* L.

Balsam cucumbers—*Momordica charantia* L.

Balsam pears—*Momordica charantia* L.

Bearberry—*Arctostaphylos uva-ursi* var. *coactilis* Fern. & Macb.

Beech—*Fagus grandiflora* Ehrh. = American beech.

Bitter root—*Apocynum androsaemifolium* L.

Blackberry—*Rubus* spp. Four species, *R. allegheniensis* Porter = Allegheny blackberry; *R. alumnus* Bailey; *R. argutus* Link. = highbush blackberry; and *R. frondosus* Bigelow = leafy-flowered blackberry are more or less common in Indiana. There are, in addition, numerous forms and varieties.

Black birch—*Betula lenta* L.

Black gum—*Nyssa sylvatica* var. *typica* Fern.

Black mustard—*Brassica nigra* (L.) Koch; *B.* juncea (L.) Czerniaew.

Black walnut—*Juglans nigra* L.

Bloodroot—*Sanguinaria canadensis* L.

Blue flag—*See* Fleur-de-lis.

Boneset—*Eupatorium perfoliatum* L.

Buckeye—*Aesculus glabra* Willd.

Buckhorn plantain—*Plantago lanceolata* L.

181

Bull thistle—*Cirsium vulgare* (Savi) Airy-Shaw
Burdock—*Arctium minus* (Hill) Bernh. = common burdock.
Butterflyweed—*Asclepias tuberosa* L.
Butternut—*Juglans cinerea* L. = white walnut.
Buttonweed—*Diodia teres* var. *setifolia* Fern. & Grisc. = rough
buttonweed.

C

Calamus—*Acorus calamus* L.
Caraway—*Carum carvi* L.
Catnip—*Nepeta cataria* L.
Chamomile—*Anthemis nobilis* L., the Roman or English chamomile, occurs wild in Indiana as does *Anthemis arvensis* L., the
field chamomile. Rayless chamomile, *Matricaria matrica-*
rioides (Less.) Porter is also found in the state, and German
chamomile, *Matricaria chamomilla* L. is cultivated here. Used
without qualification and referring to a wild plant, the name
chamomile probably means *Anthemis nobilis.* I have designated it as such in the various recipes, but all of the above
plants probably possess similar medicinal properties and may
be used interchangeably.
Chestnut—*Castanea dentata* (Marsh.) Borkh.
Chickweed—*Stellaria media* (L.) Cyril.
Chicory—*Chicorium intybus* L.
Chokecherry—*Prunus virginiana* L.
Clover—Used with qualification, the word clover may refer to either
white clover, *Trifolium repens* L., or red clover, *Trifolium pra-*
tense L. Both are common in Indiana, and the flowers of both
have similar medicinal reputations.
Cocklebur—Three species occur in Indiana. *Xanthium spinosum*
L., the spiny cocklebur, is not common but has been reported
from some of the southern counties. *Xanthium pennsylvani-*
cum Wallr., the smooth-body cocklebur, and *Xanthium itali-*
cum Moretti, the hairy-body cocklebur, both occur frequently
in moist places throughout the state.
Comfrey—*Symphytum officinale* L.
Common goldenrod—*See* Goldenrod.
Coralroot—*Corallorrhiza odontorhiza* Nutt. = late coralroot.
Corn—*Zea mays* L.
Cow parsnip—*Heracleum lanatum* Michx.
Crab apple—*Malus* spp.
Crabgrass—*Digitaria sanguinalis* (L.) Scop.
Cranesbill—*Geranium maculatum* L.
Crawley root—*Corallorrhiza odontorhiza* Nutt.

D

Dandelion—*Taraxacum officinale* Web.

Deadly nightshade—*Atropa belladonna* L.

Devil's tongue—*Sansevieria* spp., probably most commonly *S. trifasciata* Prain = mother-in-law's tongue.

Digitalis—*Digitalis purpurea* L.

Dill—*Anethum graveolens* L.

Dittany—*Cunila origanoides* (L.) Britt.

Dock—Several species are relatively common in the state. *Rumex altissimus* Wood = pale dock; *R. verticillatus* L. = swamp dock; *R. triangulivalvis* (Danser) Rech. f. = ordinarily taken for pale dock; *R. brittanica* L. = great water dock; *R. crispus* L. = curly dock; and *R. obtusifolius* L. = buntleaf dock.

Dogfennel—*Anthemis cotula* L. = mayweed.

Dogwood—*Cornus florida* L.

E

Elder—*Sambucus canadensis* L. = American elder or elderberry.

Elecampane—*Inula helenium* L.

Elm—*Ulmus americana* L. = American elm.

English plantain—*Plantago lanceolata* L.

F

Feverfew—*Chrysanthemum parthenium* (L.) Bernh.

Feverweed—*See* Feverfew.

Flax—*Linum usitatissimum* L.

Fleur-de-lis—The most common wild iris in Indiana is the Virginia iris, *Iris virginica* var. *shrevei* (Small) E. Anderson. It is often confused with the true fleur-de-lis or blue flag, *Iris versicolor* L. which may occur in northern Indiana.

Fluxweed—*Euphorbia supina* Raf.

Foxglove—*Digitalis purpurea* L.

G

Gentian—*Gentiana quinquefolia* var. *occidentalis* (Gray) Hitchc.

Ginseng—*Panax quinquefolius* L.

Goldenrod—More than two-dozen species of *Solidago* have been reported in Indiana. Many of them are widely distributed throughout the state. Some of the species are quite difficult to identify with certainty.

Goldenseal—*Hydrastis canadensis* L.

Ground ivy—*Glechoma hederacea* L. = large-flower ground ivy; *G. hederacea* var. *parviflora* (Benth.) House = small-flower ground ivy. The latter variety is much more common in Indiana.

H

Hawthorn—Several dozen species of *Crataegus* occur in Indiana.

Heal-all—*Prunella vulgaris* L. or selfheal is established in Indiana, but even more common is *Prunella vulgaris* var. *lanceolata* (Bart.) Fern., the American selfheal.

Hemlock—*Tsuga canadensis* (L.) Carr. = Eastern hemlock.

Honeylocust—*Gleditsia triacanthos* L.

Houseleek—*Sempervivum tectorum* L.

Hop-hornbeam—*Ostrya virginiana* (Mill.) K. Koch.

Hops—*Humulus americanus* Nutt. is the native species widely distributed in Indiana. *Humulus lupulus* L. is the cultivated Eurasian species.

Horehound—*Marrubium vulgare* L.

Horsebalm—*Collinsonia canadensis* L.

Horse chestnut—*Aesculus hippocastanum* L.

Horsemint—*Monarda punctata* var. *villicaulis* Pennell.

Horseradish—*Armoracia rusticana* Gaertn.

Horse weed—*Erigeron canadense* L.

Huckleberry—*Gaylussacia baccata* (Wangenh.) K. Koch.

I

Indiana rhubarb—*Rheum emodi* Wall., *R. webbianum* Royle, and related *Rheum* species. These are not native to Indiana but to India, Pakistan, and Nepal. Indian rhubarb is used for its laxative properties. Compare rhubarb (garden rhubarb) which is widely cultivated in the state. It is used for its astringent effect.

Indian turnip—*Arisaema triphyllum* (L.) Schott.

Ironweed—Indiana has only three species but they are difficult to distinguish because of intergrading forms. They are: *Veronia altissima* Nutt., *V. fasciculata* Michx., and *V. missurica* Raf.

Ironwood—*Ostrya virginiana* (Mill.) K. Koch.

J

Jack-in-the-pulpit—*Arisaema triphyllum* (L.) Schott.

Jack oak—*Quercus ellipsoidalis* E. J. Hill. Caution. In the field this tree is easily confused with the scarlet oak, *Q. coccinea* Muench., or the black oak, *Q. velutina* Lam.

Jewelweed—*Impatiens biflora* Walt. = spotted touch-me-not; *I. pallida* Nutt. = pale touch-me-not.

Jimson weed—*Datura stramonium* L.

Job's tears—*Coix lachryma-jobi* L.

Joe-pye-weed—Three species are found in Indiana. Green-stem joe-pye-weed is *Eupatorium purpureum* L. It occurs throughout the state. Purple-stem joe-pye-weed, *E. fistulosum* Barratt, is found primarily in the southern half while spotted-stem joe-pye-weed, *E. maculatum* L. grows mainly in the lake area. The medicinal properties of all three species are probably similar.

K
Knot grass—*Polygonum aviculare* L.

L
Ladyslipper—Used without qualification, the term ladyslipper could refer to several native Indiana species. *Cypripedium reginae* Walt. is the showy ladyslipper; *C. candidum* Muhl. *is the white ladyslipper; C. calceolus* var. *pubescens* (Willd.) Correll designates the yellow ladyslipper; and *C. acaule* Ait. is the pink ladyslipper.

Lamb's quarters—*Chenopodium album* L.

Lavender—*Lavandula angustifolia* Mill.

Licorice—*Glycyrrhiza glabra* L. and related varieties.

Liverwort—Two species of the genus *Hepatica* are reported from Indiana: *H. acutiloba* DC. = sharplobe hepatica; *H. americana* (DC.) Ker. = roundlobe hepatica.

Lobelia—*Lobelia inflata* L.

Lovage—*Levisticum officinale* W. D. J. Koch.

M
Mare's tail—*Erigeron canadense* L.

Marihuana—*Cannabis sativa* L.

Mayapple—*Podophyllum peltatum* L.

Milk purslane—*Euphorbia supina* Raf.

Milkweed—*Asclepias syriaca* L.

Mullein—*Verbascum thapsus* L.

Mustard—*Brassica nigra* (L.) Koch or *B. juncea* (L.) Czerniaew = black or brown mustard; *B. hirta* Moench = white or yellow mustard. The latter species is not considered to be established as a wild plant in Indiana.

N
Narrow dock—*Rumex crispus* L.

Nettle—*Urtica dioica* L., the European nettle, is rare in Indiana. *U. procera* Muhl. in Willd., known as the tall nettle, is, on the other hand, widely distributed. It is often confused with the former species.

Nightshade—Used without further qualification, nightshade ordinarily designates the common or black nightshade, *Solanum nigrum* L. However, the bitter nightshade, *Solanum dulcumara* L., is rather frequent in the lake area, and some informants may actually be referring to this species.

Northern prickly ash—*Zanthoxylum americanum* Mill.

Oak—*Quercus* spp. More than a dozen species of *Quercus* are found in Indiana. One of the most common is the white oak, *Q. alba* L.

Old-field balsam—*Gnaphalium obtusifolium* L. = sweet life everlasting.

Oswego tea—*Monarda didyma* L.

P

Peach—*Prunus persica* (L.) Stokes

Pennyroyal—*Hedeoma pulegioides* (L.) Pers.

Peppermint—*Mentha piperita* L.

Plantain—The so-called common plantain, *Plantago major* L., is rare in Indiana. Rugel plantain, *P. rugelii* Decne., is probably the most common species, but half-a-dozen others occur with some frequency. All are probably similar in their medicinal properties.

Pleurisy root—*Asclepias tuberosa* L.

Poison ivy—*Toxicodendron radicans* (L.) Kuntze. The plant is also known as *Rhus radicans* L.

Poison sumac—*Toxicodendron vernix* (L.) Kuntze. The plant is also known as *Rhus vernix* L.

Poke—*Phytolacca americana* L.

Prickly nettle—*See* Nettle.

Prostrate spurge—*Euphorbia supina* Raf.

Q

Queen-of-the-meadow—*Eupatorium purpureum* L. See also Joe-pye-weed.

R

Ragweed—*Ambrosia elatior* L.

Rattlesnake (rattlesnake's) master—Several plants growing in Indiana have been so designated. *Liatris scariosa* (L.) Willd. and *L. squarrosa* Willd. are perhaps the best possibilities. *Agave virginica* L., the false aloe, is another likely candidate. Since none is effective against rattlesnake bite, the exact identity is not of great importance.

Red alder—*See* Swamp alder.

Red clover—*Trifolium pratense* L.

Red sumac—*Rhus glabra* L.

Rhubarb—*Rheum rhaponticum* L. = garden rhubarb.

Rose—The pasture rose, *Rosa carolina* L., is the most common wild rose in the state.

Rosemary—*Rosmarinus officinalis* L.

Rue—*Ruta graveolens* L. = garden rue.

S

Sage—*Salvia officinalis* L.

Sarsaparilla—Authentic sarsaparilla is obtained from several species of *Similax* growing in Central and South America. In Indiana, so-called wild sarsaparilla, *Aralia nudicaulis* L., has been frequently substituted for it.

Sassafras—*Sassafras albidum* (Nutt.) Nees.

Sedge or Sedge grass—*Carex* species. About 2000 different ones occur in Indiana.

Sedum—Probably most often refers to the cultivated *Sedum acre* L.

Senna—*Cassia acutifolia* Del. = Alexandria senna; *C. angustifolia* Vahl = Tinnevelly senna.

Shagbark hickory—*Carya ovata* (Mill.) K. Koch.

Sheep sorrel—Two very different species are often designated by this same common name. They may be differentiated on the basis of their flower colors. *Oxalis stricta* L. has yellow flowers; *Rumex acetosella* L. has red flowers.

Shoo-fly—*Nicandra physalodes* (L.) Pers.

Silkweed—*Asclepias syriaca* L.

Skunk cabbage—*Symplocarpus foetidus* (L.) Nutt.

Slippery elm—*Ulmus fulva* Michx.

Smartweed—*Polygonum punctatum* Ell. = water smartweed.

Smooth sumac—*Rhus glabra* L.

Snakeroot—The number of different snakeroots is legion. Canada snakeroot (*Asarum canadense* L.), Virginia snakeroot (*Aristolochia serpentaria* L.), and button-snakeroot (*Eryngium yuccaefolium* Michx.) all occur in the state.

Snakeweed—*Aristolochia serpentaria* L. = Virginia snakeroot or serpentaria.

Solomon's seal—*Polygonatum pubescens* (Willd.) Pursh = hairy Solomon's seal; *P. biflorum* (Walt.) Ell. (complex) = smooth Solomon's seal.

Sour dock—*Rumex crispus* L.

Spearmint—*Mentha spicata* L.

Spicebush—*Benzoin aestivale* (L.) Nees.

Spicewood—*Benzoin aestivale* (L.) Nees.

Spikenard—*Aralia racemosa* L.

Spotted spurge—*Euphorbia supina* Raf.

Spruce—*Picea* spp. All of the *Picea* species in Indiana are introduced; none is native to the state.

Stargrass—*Aletris farinosa* L. = unicorn root.

Starweed—*Stellaria media* (L.) Cyr.

Stonecrop—*Sedum* spp. (q.v.).

Stoneroot—*Collinsonia canadensis* L.

Stramonium—*Datura stramonium* L.

Sugar maple—*Acer saccharum* Marsh.

Sumac—Used without qualification, this refers to *Rhus glabra* L., the smooth or scarlet sumac. However, several other species and hybrids with red berries occur in Indiana. These include *R. typhina* L., the staghorn sumac, *R. copallina* L., the shining sumac, and *X Rhus pulvinata* Greene (*Rhus glabra X typhina*).

Summer savory—*Satureja hortensis* L.

Swamp alder—The true red alder or swamp alder, *Alnus rubra* Bong., is not found in Indiana. Informants probably used the speckled alder, *A. incana* var. *americana* Regel., or the hazel alder, *A. rugosa* (Ehrh.) Spreng. Both species favor moist habitats.

Sweet anise—*Osmorhiza longistylis* (Torr.) DC.

Sweet cicely—*Osmorhiza claytoni* (Michx.) Clarke.

Sweet life everlasting—*Gnaphalium obtusifolium* L. = old-field balsam

Sweet wormwood—*Artemesia annua* L.

Sycamore—*Platanus occidentalis* L.

T

Thyme—*Thymus vulgaris* L.

Tobacco—*Nicotiana tabacum* L.

Touch-me-not—*See* Jewelweed.

Trumpet weed—*Eupatorium purpurem* L.; *E. fistulosum* Barratt; and *E. maculatum* L. See comments under Joe-pye-weed.

Tulip tree—*Liriodendron tulipifera* L.

U

Unicorn root—*Aletris farinosa* L. = stargrass.

V

Valerian—*Valeriana officinalis* L.

Vermifuge—*Chenopodium ambrosiodes* var. *anthelminticum* (L.) Gray = wormseed.

Violet—*Viola* spp. *Viola sororia* Willd., the downy blue violet, is the most common of the two-dozen species in Indiana.

W

Watercress—*Nasturtium officinale* R. Br.

Wheat—*Triticum aestivum* L.

White ash—*Fraxinus americana* L.

White Easter lily—*Lilium longiflorum* var. *eximium* (Courtois) Bak. Several other cultivated varieties are commonly referred to as Easter lilies.

White maple—*Acer saccharinum* L.

White mustard—*Brassica alba* (L.) Hook. f.

White oak—*Quercus alba* L.

White sassafras—A form of *Sassafras albidum* (Nutt.) Nees. with whitish root bark, and with smooth leaves, buds, and young twigs. Possibly *S. albidum* var. *molle* (Raf.) Fern.

White snakeroot—*Eupatorium rugosum* Houtt.

White walnut—*Juglans cinerea* L. = butternut.

Wild black cherry—*Prunus serotina* Ehrh.

Wild celery—*Apium graveolens* L.

Wild cherry—*Prunus serotina* Ehrh. = black cherry or wild black cherry.

Wild daisy—The one most frequently found in Indiana is the oxeye daisy, *Chrysanthemum leucanthemum* var. *pinnatifidum* Lecoq & Lamotte.

Wild garlic—Several species occur: *Allium vineale* L. = crow garlic and *A. canadense* L. = meadow garlic. In addition to these two native species, *A. sativum* L., an escaped form of the cultivated garlic, is found growing wild in Indiana.

Wild geranium—*Geranium maculatum* L.

Wild ginger—*Asarum canadense* L. = Canada wild ginger; also *A. reflexum* Bickn. = curly wild ginger.

Wild lettuce—*Lactuca scariola* L. = prickly lettuce.

Wild mint—This generic designation refers to any or all of the various species of *Blephilia*, *Monarda*, and *Pycnanthemum* found in the state.

Wild mustard—*Brassica kaber* var. *pinnatifida* (Stokes) Wheeler.

Wild onion—*Allium cernuum* Roth. = nodding onion; *A. stellatum* Ker.

Wild peppermint—*Mentha piperita* L. This is ordinary peppermint that has escaped cultivation.

Wild poplar—*Liriodendron tulipifera* L.

Wild senna—*Cassia hebecarpa* Fern.

Wild strawberry—*Fragaria virginiana* Duch.

Wild touch-me-not—*See* Jewelweed.

Willow—*Salix* spp. About twenty species occur in Indiana.

Witch hazel—*Hamamelis virginiana* L.

Wormroot—*Spigelia marilandica* L. = pinkroot.

Wormseed—*Chenopodium ambrosioides* var. antheminticum (L.) Gray.

Wormwood—*Artemesia absinthium* L. = common wormwood.

Y

Yarrow—*Achillea millefolium* L.

Yellow birch—*Betula lutea* var. *macrolepis* Fern.

Yellow dock—*Rumex crispus* L.

Yellow root—*Hydrastis canadensis* L.

Yellow-flowered sorrel—*Oxalis stricta* L. = yellow wood sorrel = sheep sorrel.

Yellow ladyslipper—*Cypripedium calceolus* var. *pubescens* (Willd.) Correll.

Suggestions for Further Reading

Persons interested in learning more about the identity and potential curative properties of drugs used as home remedies have a great abundance of literature at their disposal. The problem is that much of it is not reliable. It is advocacy literature designed to sell a product, not to provide an accurate insight into the pros and cons of herbs and other simple medicaments. To read it without a proper guide is like journeying through the land of Oz without a yellow brick road. Without such a guide, the reader will be exposed to some fantastic things, but many will bear little resemblance to reality.

The following brief annotated bibliography will serve as a guide to just a few of the reliable books devoted to this fascinating field. Many of them contain useful references that will allow the reader access to the vast and important periodical literature on drugs and their use. The order of listing is according to the type of subject matter: Comprehensive, Pharmacognosy (Natural Drugs), Pharmacology and Therapeutics, Toxicology, and Botany. Naturally, there is some overlap among the categories.

Comprehensive

Included in this classification are works that cover all aspects of the entire field of drugs. Unfortunately, there is no up-to-date American reference in this category.

The Dispensatory of the United States of America, twenty-fifth edition; Arthur Osol and George E. Farrar, Jr.; J. B. Lippincott Company, Philadelphia, 1955, 2,139 pages.

This useful work ceased publication in its present form with the twenty-fifth edition. Previous editions, such as the twenty-fourth (1947) and the twenty-third (1943) are also very useful, especially for some of the older remedies.

Martindale: The Extra Pharmacopoeia, twenty-eighth edition; James E. F. Reynolds, editor; The Pharmaceutical Press, London, 1982, 2,025 pages.

Although of British origin, this is a most useful volume. Providing comprehensive coverage of practically all medicinal substances, it is replete with references to the literature. Highly recommended.

Pharmacognosy (Natural Drugs)

Many of the recommended home remedies are obtained from plants or animals; consequently, they are most thoroughly discussed in works on pharmacognosy.

A Dictionary of Terms in Pharmacognosy; George M. Hocking; Charles C Thomas, Springfield, Illinois, 1955, 284 pages.
This is most useful to anyone attempting to understand the nomenclature of this complex field.

Medical Botany; Walter H. Lewis and Memory P.F. Elvin-Lewis; John Wiley & Sons, New York, 1977, 515 pages.
A helpful compilation of botanical drugs and their uses.

Encyclopedia of Common Natural Ingredients Used in Food, Drugs and Cosmetics; Albert Y. Leung; John Wiley & Sons, New York, 1980, 409 pages.
Provides detailed coverage, in monographic fashion, on the botany, chemistry, and pharmacology of vegetable drugs and spices. Many good references.

Herbs: An Indexed Bibliography, 1971–1980; James E. Simon, Alena F. Chadwick, and Lyle E. Craker; Archer Books, Hamden, Connecticut, 1984, 770 pages.
A listing of thousands of references to the chemistry, botany, bionomics, horticulture, production ecology, culinary studies, pharmacology, and perfumery of herbs.

The Honest Herbal; Varro E. Tyler; George F. Stickley Company, Philadelphia, 1982, 263 pages.
A critical evaluation of the safety and efficacy of more than 100 of the most widely used herbs. Hundreds of pertinent references.

Pharmacognosy, eighth edition; Varro E. Tyler, Lynn R. Brady, and James E. Robbers; Lea & Febiger, Philadelphia, 1981, 520 pages.
The standard text and reference book in the field. In addition to coverage of the conventional drugs, it contains a chapter on "Herbs and Health Foods" as well as one on "Poisonous Plants."

Pharmacology and Therapeutics

Because of the complexity of the field of pharmacology, modern texts and reference books, to retain a manageable size, now restrict their coverage to a limited number of drugs selected on the basis of their widespread use and effectiveness. This renders the books without value in providing information on most of the products that have been, and continue to be, widely used as folk medicines. Because no modern, comprehensive encyclopedia of pharmacology exists, the interested reader is forced to utilize older books to obtain even meager pharmacological information about herbal remedies and related products.

A Manual of Pharmacology, eighth edition; Torald Sollman; W. B. Saunders Company, Philadelphia, 1957, 1,535 pages.
Without question the best pharmacology book ever written, this volume published nearly thirty years ago is now seriously dated in many respects. However, in its discussion of common products used as home remedies, it is still the best available. Even at the time of publication, the field was so vast that the publishers were forced to restrict the literature references to those appearing since January 1, 1940. For the earlier references, it is necessary to consult the bibliographies in the fifth (1936) and the sixth (1942) editions as well.

Sollman Bibliographies; The Dow Chemical Company, Midland, Michigan, and Indianapolis, no date.
To facilitate use, this combined reprint of all the different bibliographies has appeared.

Handbook of Nonprescription Drugs, seventh edition; American Pharmaceutical Association, Washington, D.C.; 1982, 682 pages.
This book devotes thirty-four chapters to the composition and therapeutic use of all the popular self-selected remedies commercially available. It contains numerous references and provides considerable information on self-treatment of various ailments.

The Merck Manual, fourteenth edition; Robert Berkow, editor-in-chief; Merck Sharp & Dohme Research Laboratories, Rahway, New Jersey, 1982, 2,578 pages.
A standard reference work on the diagnosis and therapy of disease.

Toxicology

A Colour Atlas of Poisonous Plants; Dietrich Frohne and Hans J. Pfänder; Wolfe Publishing Ltd., London, 1984, 291 pages.

A beautifully illustrated, up-to-date reference on plants that are, or are thought to be, poisonous. Contains an extensive bibliography.

Clinical Toxicology of Commercial Products, fifth edition; Robert E. Gosselin, Roger P. Smith, and Harold C. Hodge; Williams & Wilkins, Baltimore, 1984, 2,000 pages.

Detailed discussion, with references, of all aspects of the poisonous character of the ingredients of most commercial products.

Botany

The classic reference in the field, and the one used in the preparation of *Hoosier Home Remedies,* is:

Flora of Indiana; Charles C. Deam, Department of Conservation, Division of Forestry, Indianapolis, 1940, 1,236 pages.

It is particularly useful in providing maps of Indiana that depict the counties, showing in which ones the various species have been collected. Also very valuable in listing the locally used common names of plants.

The Vascular Plants of Indiana; A Computer Based Checklist; Theodore J. Crovello, Clifton A. Keller, and John T. Kartesz; The American Midland Naturalist and University of Notre Dame Press, Notre Dame, 1983, 136 pages.

A recent inventory, using modern botanical nomenclature, of all plant species known in Indiana. Supplements but does not replace Deam.

Index

Puffball, 16, 18
Pumpkin Seeds, 101, 103, 104, 171, 172
Puncture (Wounds), 173, 175, 176, 177
Purgative, 15, 51, 52, 89
Purge, 52
Purifiers, 19–26, 109
Pycnanthemum spp., 48, 149, 154, 155

Queen Elizabeth II, 49
Queen-of-the-Meadow, 45, 103, 104, 107
Quercus alba, 57
Quercus ellipsoidalis, 100
Quercus spp., 18
Quinine, 45, 107
Quinones, 141

Rabid, 129
Rabies, 128–29
Ragweed, 70
Raisin(s), 6, 34, 52, 118, 163, 164
Rash(es), 99, 108, 109, 123, 124, 125, 126, 127, 128, 133, 134
    Allergic, 93
Rats, 157
Rattlesnake, 8
    Bite, 137
Rattlesnake Master, 137
Red Alder, 93
Red Clover, 22, 35, 133
Redness (Skin), 134
Red Sumac, 100, 114
Repellant(s)
    Chigger, 97, 98
    Insect, 98–99
Respiratory, 13
    Infection, 60
Rest, 62
Rheumatism, 2, 3, 5–11
Rheum emodi, 71
Rheum rhaponticum, 70, 71, 96, 133
Rheum webbianum, 71
Rhubarb (Root)
    Garden, 70, 71, 72
    Indian, 71, 72
Rhubarb (Stock), 96, 133, 134, 135

Rhus glabra, 12, 100, 114, 159
Ringworm, 129–31
Root Beer, 25
Rosa spp., 19
Rose Hips, 19
Rosemary, 87
Rosewater, 177, 179
Rosin, 59, 64, 136, 166, 176, 179
Rosmarinus officinalis, 87
Rub, 146, 147
Rubefacient(s), 89, 149, 150
Rubus spp., 68
Rue, 99
Rumex acetosella, 23, 154
Rumex crispus, 20, 24, 35, 163
Rumex spp., 95, 116, 130, 131
Ruta graveolens, 99
Rye Meal, 122

Sabatia angularis, 107
Safrole, 25, 160
Sage, 45, 83, 87, 108, 109, 114, 143, 145, 154, 156
Saleratus, 100
Salicin (salicyl alcohol gluco-side), 10, 89
Salicylates, 10, 89
Saliva, 129, 130, 140, 141, 162
Salix spp., 9, 88, 169
Salt, 17, 18, 27, 36, 45, 55, 69, 74, 79, 80, 97, 111, 112, 114, 125, 127, 135, 136, 141, 142, 143, 144, 145, 148, 149, 161, 162, 164, 178
Salt Herring, 171
Saltpeter, 9, 13
Salt Pork, 74, 140, 141, 176
Salts, 89
Salve(s), 135
    Apple, 179
    Balm of Gilead Buds, 30
    Beeswax, 64, 179
    Black Birch, 6, 10
    Carrots, 18
    Chamomile, 36
    Houseleek, 95
    Jimson Weed, 90